Thirry A. Fole

W9-AKD-741

Praise for

The Vegetarian Revolution

"*The Vegetarian Revolution* is a fact, not fiction. It is a fact of life. It is a choice that hundreds of people are making every day."

—Dr. Michael Fox, Vice President of
The Humane Society of the United States

"*The Vegetarian Revolution* is not only fascinating, fun and engrossing, it has the potential—if its message is heeded—to literally save the world. This is a must read for everyone concerned about the fate of our planet and what we can do to save it."

—Lewis Regenstein, author of *Replenishing The Earth* and President of The Interfaith Council for the Protection of Animals and Nature

"Like a revolutionary idea whose time has come, Giorgio Cerquetti's *The Vegetarian Revolution* is destined to change hearts, minds and eating habits throughout the world."

—Rynn Berry, author of *Famous Vegetarians and Their Favorite Recipes* and *Food for the Gods: Vegetarianism and the World's Religions*

SMYRNA PUBLIC LIBRARY

DISCARD

DISCARD

THE VEGETARIAN REVOLUTION

SMYRNA PUBLIC LIBRARY

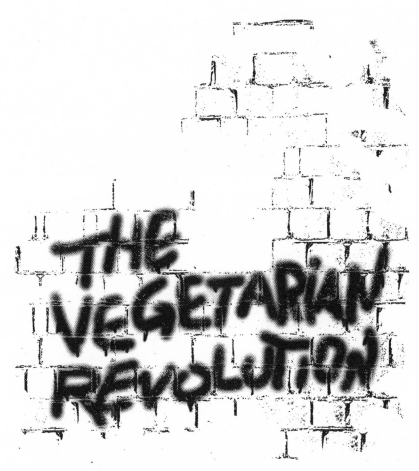

Giorgio Cerquetti

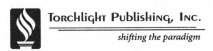

Torchlight Publishing, Inc.

shifting the paradigm

Copyright © 1997 by Giorgio Cerquetti

All rights reserved. No part of this book may be reproduced, stored in a retrieval system, or transmitted in any form, by any means, including mechanical, electronic, photocopying, recording, or otherwise, without prior written consent of the publisher.

First Printing 1997

Design by Stewart Cannon / Logo Loco Graphics
Cover design by Jean Greisser and Stewart Cannon
Printed in the United States of America

Published simultaneously in The United States of America and Canada by Torchlight Publishing

Library of Congress Cataloging-in-Publishing Data
Cerquetti, Giorgio 1946—
    The vegetarian revolution / by Giorgio Cerquetti,

          p.   cm.
    ISBN 1-887089-00-4
    1.Vegetarian cookery.   2. Vegetarianism..   I. Title.

    TX837.C384   1997   97-19203
    641.5'636--dc21

Attention Colleges, Universities, Corporations, Associations and Professional Organizations: *The Vegetarian Revolution* is available at special discounts for bulk purchases for promotions, premiums, fund-raising or educational use. Special books, booklets, or excerpts can be created to suit your specific needs.

For more information contact the Publisher

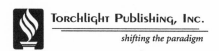
ΤσrchliqhT Publishing, Inc.
shifting the paradigm

PO Box 52 Badger CA 93603
Email: Torchlight@compuserve.com
1-888-TorchLt toll free

Dedication

This book is dedicated to open-minded FREE SPIRITS with good hearts and a global vision. May this humble contribution to an evolving popular culture, based on eternal values of love, respect and cooperation, touch as many sincere hearts as possible with the universal message of vegetarianism.

The political strategy of "divide and conquer" has caused pain and suffering long enough; an authoritarian culture has made mankind weak. We can regain our strength and joy if we choose to unite with sincere and sensitive people to fearlessly share the Earth with LOVE. Meditate on this inspiring vision; your immediate action can save the lives of billions of innocent creatures killed every year to feed other humans like us. Our valid hope for a better future is that mankind will become finally aware that every-BODY—human and nonhuman—has the same right to exist on this planet.

After centuries of devastating wars and vicious fights for control, the major issue of the next millennium will be nonviolence—the remarkable achievement of harmony and peace on the international level, beginning with personal responsibility in the relationships we each have daily to life and death decisions involving other living beings. So let's remove, once and for all, discriminations and misconceptions from our minds and include animals in the Great Planetarian Family. Remember, life is a divine gift!

Love God, love people, love animals—be happy and enjoy the unity of all life.

Special Thanks

To all the active vegetarian groups and gentle individuals that responded to our request for original recipes. A special thanks to Rynn Berry and Yamuna Devi for providing selected recipes of some great vegetarians. Rynn Berry is a renowned scholar and author of *Famous Vegetarians*; we recommend everybody read his excellent book. Thanks to Bharat dasa for his wonderful cartoon art creations used throughout this book. My deep gratitude goes to Kay Vontillius for her spiritual support.

Table of Contents

Recipe List

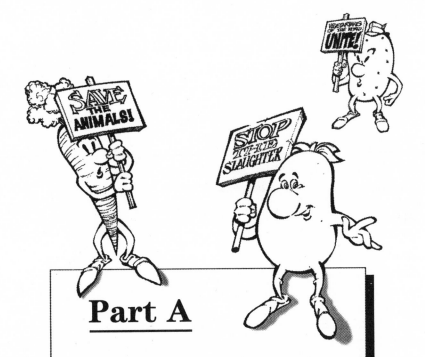

Part A

The Vegetarian Revolution

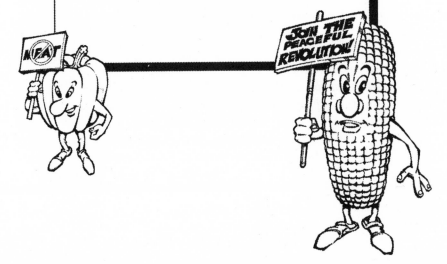

There is one thing stronger
than all the armies of the world
and that is an idea
whose time has come.

—Victor Hugo

The most peaceful, nonviolent and global REVOLUTION in history is now emerging—to cease killing animals and commence teaching LOVE and respect for ALL LIFE.

**DEAR FRIENDS, PLEASE JOIN THIS
PEACEFUL REVOLUTION...**

I have no doubt that it is part of the destiny of
the human race in its gradual development to
leave off the eating of animals, as surely as
the savage tribes have left off eating each other
when they came in contact with the more civilized.

—Henry David Thoreau

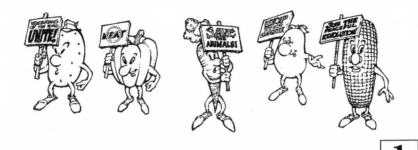

Join The Revolution

Finally, the time of VEGETARIANISM has come!

Since the Sixties, hundreds of good books have been written about vegetarianism. Thousands of successful restaurants throughout the world are serving tasty and nutritious, meat-free meals to millions of people who appreciate the many values of a healthy and natural vegetarian diet. So what is the need of another book?

The Vegetarian Revolution is a call to arms...arms that protect by embracing all sentient beings in their care. It allows those not so inclined to reading an easy reference to gain good "one-liners" that establish the commonsense basis for vegetarianism and arguments in its defense. Herein also is a simple yet powerful plea to take up a way of life that is by its nature compassionate: mercy to animals and manifest concern for the hunger daily found in one's immediate contact with less fortunate human beings. A concise presentation for wide distribution to incite change, along with recipes to make that change very pleasant—this is the purpose of *The Vegetarian Revolution*.

The word *vegetarian* was coined by the founders of the British Vegetarian Society in 1842. Etymologically, *vegetarian* comes from the Latin word *vegetus,* meaning "whole, fresh, alive." *Homo Vegetus* means, literally, a physically and mentally healthy, vigorous person. The original meaning of this word was broader in its cultural context and meant more than just a meat-free diet or ordinary improvement in cooking habits.

A vegetarian who abstains from any food of animal origin (such as milk and honey) and other animal products is called a *vegan.* Vegetarianism is a viable alternative for those who are entirely convinced that the violent characteristics related to animal eating are unacceptable but find *veganism* extreme, personally and/or socially. Domesticating animals for their gifts doesn't necessarily involve their suffering, although most modern industries are quite guilty of animal cruelty. The vegetarian life style is one of balance between the spiritual and social ways of life.

After many years of constant "underground" growth, the vegetarian movement is no longer just the preserve of an avant-garde elite, who were often presented by mainstream media as a fanatical subculture. On the contrary, vegetarianism is a very visible alternative now embraced by millions of people all over the world. Slaughterhouses and drug companies (and those who profit by their industries) quake at the prospect of this compassionate cultural renaissance. But now is the time for this graceful transformation.

We can continue reshaping the world—starting from within our own homes, from within our own kitchens, within our own selves. We must set a positive ethical example for our families and friends. We should express openly our positive commitment to transform the planet and invite everyone we meet to remove flesh and blood from their cook pots and serving dishes. This senseless killing of animals devastates our environment, our bodies and our minds.

Today's Meat Is Nothing Like Primitive Meat

"Don't try to justify your meat-eating habit by making up your nutritional roots!" admonished Dr. Paavo Airola. "Unless your roots are in Polar Regions, your ancestors were not heavy meat-eaters. Excessive meat-eating is a very recent phenomenon, both in the United States and elsewhere in the world. Until just a few generations ago, meat was eaten only occasionally, mostly on weekends and holidays. This was true in European countries as well as in the United States. It is safe to say that 99% of all Americans have nutritional roots in low-animal-protein backgrounds, and thus will achieve better health on such a diet."

Often meat eaters bring out the argument that our ancestors were carnivorous. Wrong! They were omnivorous, not carnivorous. Our ancestors had very large molars with small incisors, unsuited to meat consumption but ideal for consuming large quantities of vegetable matter. As zoologist Desmond Morris observes in his book *The Naked Ape*, "It could be argued that since our primate ancestors had to make do without a major meat component in their diets, we should be able to do the same. We were driven to become flesh eaters only by environmental circumstances, and now that we have the environment under control, with elaborately cultivated crops at our disposal, we might be expected to return to our ancient primate feeding patterns."

In his book *Why We Don't Eat Meat*, Peter Cox, former Chief Executive of the powerful Vegetarian Society of The United Kingdom, explains the risks today's meat eaters are taking:

> Another big difference between our ancestors' diet and the food we eat today is not just in the quantity of meat consumed, but also its quality. Modern food animals are bred to be fat. The carcass of a slaughtered animal can easily be thirty percent or more fat. But the sort of animal that primitive people hunted was a wild animal. It had, on average, only 3.9 percent fat on its carcass. So, today, even if we cut our meat consumption back to the greatly reduced amount that our ancestors consumed, we will still be taking in seven times more fat!
>
> Primitive meat had five times more polyunsaturated fat than today's meat does, which is high in saturated fat but much lower in polyunsaturated fat. Our ancestral diet had only one-sixth the amount of sodium (salt) that the modern diet contains. Because fresh food comprised such an important part of the diet, the primitive diet was much, much richer in natural vita-

mins. For example, there would have been nearly nine times as much Vitamin C in the primitive diet, twice as much fiber and three times as much total polyunsaturated fat. The fact is that in terms of quantity and quality, today's meat is nothing like the primitive food that our ancestors would occasionally eat. In evolutionary terms, the meat we eat today is a new food for us. This means that we are actually conducting a huge experiment on our own bodies. And so far the results don't look good.

All You Need Is Love

"Love all of God's creation, the whole and every grain of sand in it. Love every leaf, every ray of God's light. Love the animals, love the plants, love everything. If you love everything, you will perceive the divine mystery in things."
—Fyodor Dostoyevsky, *The Brothers Karamazov*

Man Is Not Carnivorous

"Man resembles no carnivorous animal at all. The orangutan is the most anthropomorphous of the ape tribe, all of which are strictly frugivorous."
—Percy Bysshe Shelley

Murder

"Flesh eating is unprovoked murder."
—Benjamin Franklin

Dead Meat

"Dead meat should be buried, not eaten."
—Chrissie Hynde, lead singer of the Pretenders
and animal rights activist

Meat Stinks

"You can shake it, bake it or broil it, but it's still the decomposing corpse of an abused animal."
—PETA, *Guide to Compassionate Living*

Death Places

"If I enter a place where meat is served, my heart is seized with sadness when I realize that once living creatures now lie silently frozen in a coffin of ice. Frigid carcasses, cruelly denied the courtesy of cremation, await to fill new burial grounds in the warmth of human stomachs. And when I smell the odor of animal's blood and baking flesh, which permeates the granules of every brick of every wall, I feel the stain of death upon that location, and I know it cannot be the place where I will rest."
—Anonymous

Factory Farmers

"Whenever people say, 'We mustn't be sentimental,' you can take it they are about to do something cruel. And if they add, 'We must be realistic,' they mean they are going to make money out of it. These slogans have a long story. After being used to justify slave traders, ruthless industrialists, and contractors who had found that the most economically 'realistic' method of cleaning a chimney was to force a small child to climb it, they have now been passed on, like an heirloom, to the factory farmers."
—Brigid Brophy, called by *Time* magazine
"the acknowledged high priestess of
British intelligentsia"

Compassion

"Compassion is the foundation of everything positive, everything good. If you carry the power of compassion to the marketplace and the dinner table, you can make your life really count."
—Rue McClanahan

Kill, Kill, Kill

Isn't man an amazing animal? He kills birds, kangaroos, deer, all kinds of cats, coyotes, beavers, groundhogs, mice, foxes and dingoes by the millions in order to protect his domestic animals and their feed. Then he kills his domestic animals by the billions and eats them. This in turn kills man by the millions, because eating all those animals leads to degenerative and fatal-health conditions like heart disease, kidney disease and cancer. So then man tortures and kills more animals to look for cures for these diseases. Elsewhere, millions of other human beings are killed by hunger and malnutrition because food they could have eaten is being used to fatten domestic animals. Meanwhile, some people are dying of sad laughter at the absurdity of man, who kills so easily and so violently, and once a year sends out cards calling for PEACE ON EARTH.

No Bloodshed

"Oh my fellow men, do not defile your bodies with sinful foods. We have corn and apples bending down the branches with their weight. There are sweet-flavored herbs and grapes swelling on the vines. There are vegetables which can be cooked and softened over the fire, nor are you denied milk or thyme-scented honey. The earth affords a lavish supply of riches of innocent foods, and offers you banquets that involve no bloodshed or slaughter; only beasts satisfy their hunger with flesh, and not even all of those, because horses, cattle, and sheep live on grass."
—Pythagoras

The idea of this book came to me a few years ago, along with a vision of a colorful, awe-inspiring, clean and healthy planet, where all living entities can harmoniously live and thrive together in peace. I felt the close advent of a new day on our green and blue globe, floating in the universe since time immemorial. Our Earth is a magnificent unit, a marvelous "starship," where we are all—rich and poor, humans and nonhumans—just temporary passengers wearing different molecular clothes (bodies). Astronaut Edgar D. Mitchell gave this beautiful and poetic description of our planet from outer space:

Earth...is a sparkling blue and white jewel,
laced with swirling veils of white,
like a small pearl in a thick sea of black mystery.
My view of our planet was a glimpse of divinity.

The most genuine, inspiring principle and existential truth is that all residents of Earth, living in different species, are interconnected. We must coexist interdependently—each living BODY has the same rights and needs. If we forget this essential point, we cannot expect lasting peace in the world.

A fundamental shift of consciousness is desperately needed to increase our universal awareness and solve the present crises of mankind. The most significant and enlightened step we can take is our choice of food. The vegetarian decision has dramatic and immediate beneficial repercussions on our personal health, the quality of the environment and the conservation of nature and all living creatures. The future of planet Earth hangs in our conscious choices. This is not a time to be apathetic but to realize we, the people, are the solution. There is still time to resolve the increasing problems threatening life on our precious planet.

A Nobel Prize Winner Speaks Out

"How can we pray to God for mercy if we ourselves have no mercy? How can we speak of rights and justice if we take an innocent creature and shed its blood? This is my protest against the conduct of the world. To be a vegetarian is to disagree. To disagree with the course of things today. I believe that as long as human beings will go on shedding the blood of animals, there will never be any peace. There is only one little step from killing animals to creating gas chambers a la Hitler and concentration camps a la Stalin; all such things are done in the name of social justice. There will be no justice as long as man will stand with a knife or with a gun and destroy those who are weaker than he is. We must make a statement against these things. Vegetarianism is my statement and I think it's a strong one."

—Isaac Bashevis Singer, Nobel Prize in literature

Be Vegetarian

"It may indeed be doubted whether butcher's meat is anywhere a necessity for life. Grain and other vegetables, with the help of milk, cheese and butter, or oil, where butter is not to be had, afford the most plentiful, the most wholesome, the most nourishing, and the most invigorating diet. Decency nowhere requires that any man should eat butcher's meat."

—Adam Smith, *The Wealth Of Nations*

You Are Not A Human Being

"O meat eater, you are a devil, not a human being. Keep not a meat eater's company. For even his company is harmful to devotion for the Lord. Believe me, friend, those who eat meat and fish and drink intoxicating drinks will all be rooted out like weeds are taken from a fertile field, and thrown down into a dark valley of death. All flesh is one, whether it be of fowl or deer or cow, and those who eat it will go straight to hell with open eyes."

—Kabir, Sufi poet

Two Seconds of Reflection

Every two seconds in the same planet where you live, work, eat and enjoy your life with your friends and relatives, a poor child starves to death.

Did you know that? Now that you know, will you do something?

The Healing Power of Food Distribution

"Then imagine the room filled with 45 to 50 people with empty bowls in front of them. For the feed cost of your steak, each of their bowls could be filled with a full cup of cooked cereal grains."
—Frances Moore Lappe´, *Diet For A Small Planet*

The food produced daily in the world is sufficient to feed everybody. The real problem of starvation is only distribution. There is not a real scarcity of anything. While in the Western Hemisphere millions of people are overeating and/or absorbed in different diets, too many people starve and suffer daily from malnutrition in less prosperous countries. An average of 60,000 people die every single day of the year as a cruel result of this social imbalance; 40,000 are poor, innocent children. We don't blame you for this deplorable situation, but you can be part of the solution. It is a fact that some are taking more than they need, while others are starving. Be aware that this tragic problem is no longer confined to the so-called third world but is spreading in many of the major cities of America. The American Dream has for some turned into a hellish nightmare. Maybe just a few blocks away from your cozy, sweet home, a mother doesn't have enough food for her children.

Either alone or with the support of compassionate friends, you can raise funds, collect the food and go out into the street or to any homeless shelter to distribute pure and healthy vegetarian food. Don't wait for the welfare system or someone else to come forward—do it yourself. Give your honest and sincere contribution to the advancement of the new human civilization. Edmund Burke said, "Nobody made a greater mistake than he who did nothing because he could only do a little." Just doing this charitable service once a week, or even once a month, can benefit many other less fortunate members of our huge human family. Most probably within your conscience the taste for this wonderful program will increase, so we suggest that you start with a group of sincere friends, a local vegetarian task force. Our organization, Vegetarians International, can give you all the assistance and support you may need to collect goods, resources and food.

The Vegetarian Revolution, with its strong cultural and ethical foundation, can heal many wounds and make us better, more loving persons. Be spiritual, start your own "Good Karma Group" now! God is kind, merciful and vegetarian. God will bless you. You will find a new energy and can rapidly build up your self -esteem. There is no more need for tears or time wasted blaming others. We need a new American diet, one that is more compassionate, more holistic and healthy—a clear vision capable of lovingly embracing all sentient beings, humans and nonhumans. Take your good share of responsibility now and become an active distributor of FREE VEGETARIAN FOOD.

Before you come up with the main question—Who is going to pay for this free food distribution to the hungry?—let's meditate on the words of two former Presidents of the United States. On October 5, 1947, in his first televised White House address, President Truman asked Americans to refrain from eating meat on Tuesday and poultry on Thursday to help stockpile grain for starving people in Europe. General Dwight D. Eisenhower made it clear on April 16, 1953: "Every gun that is made, every sharp warship launched, every rocket fired signifies, in a final sense, a theft from those who hunger and are not fed, those who are cold and are not clothed."

This book's profits will support feeding of the homeless in the USA and needy people in India and other countries. A simple suggestion: if you meet a poor person starving in the street, don't wait for institutions or the government—do something yourself; buy some food, offer it to God and help a human being to survive another day. When we peacefully help another human being, our heart fills up with pleasure and unconditional love and it is easier to perceive that we are all ONE GREAT LOVING FAMILY.

Unfortunately, it looks like the number of starving people in the world is going to increase in the next few years. Political violence, epidemic diseases, natural calamities and economic recession are hitting millions. Generous and intelligent people like you are desperately needed to relieve some of the pain and suffering. Please distribute copies of this book and help this project by spreading these ideas to other caring people. Act now! Give them to your neighbors, your friends, your schoolmates, your teachers, your colleagues and even to unknown people. Leave them around in bus stops, schools, airports, hospitals, jails and any place where people are waiting. This reading can change their life, generate a moral aversion to flesh eating and finally make this wonderful and divine planet a better place for everybody to live, human and nonhuman alike.

We need a new culture that goes beyond the current fragmented view of the universe. The realization of the unity of all life manifesting in different species will allow the society to develop very quickly toward the Garden of Eden we all dream of.

The time is NOW. Don't hesitate. Stop the useless killing of innocent animals. Today you are welcomed to join the exalted company of such great souls as Krishna, King David, Buddha, Jesus, Mohammed, Mahavira, Pythagoras, Socrates, Plato, King Ashoka, Plutarch, Clement of Alexandria, St. Francis, Leonardo da Vinci, Montaigne, Akbar, Jon Milton, Sir Isaac Newton, Emanuel Swedenborg, Voltaire, Benjamin Franklin, Jean Jacques Rousseau, Lamartine, Percy Bysshe Shelley, Ralph Waldo Emerson, Henry David Thoreau, Leo Tolstoy, George Bernard Shaw, Franz Kafka, Annie Besant, Rabindranath Tagore, Mahatma Gandhi, Albert Schweitzer, Albert Einstein, Bhaktivedanta Swami Prabhupada, Dr. John Harvey Kellogg, Nobel Prize author Isaac Bashevis Singer and many other great souls.

Remember, most of mankind for most of human history has lived on vegetarian or near-vegetarian diets. And much of the world still follows this healthy diet.

I am very optimistic about the future expansion of vegetarianism. What's happening now is just the beginning of a widespread, international VEGETARIAN REVOLUTION. Don't buy a weapon. Don't run to the streets or hide in the mountains. This is a special revolution—totally different from similar attempts of the past—that combines spiritual growth, loving compassion and a dynamic attitude for social service. This movement is completely innocent, peaceful, nonviolent, open-minded and brilliant as the sun. It is an awakening that starts within yourself and doesn't harm any-BODY at all.

Lift your eyes from the darkness of ignorance—awareness, love, forgiveness and compassion are the "Real Solution"! We are very close to an evolution in consciousness. Probably some of you already feel that it's coming…that it's close at hand. Our greatest potential is in educating, inspiring and uniting all sentient living beings of the planet.

Humanity has already taken up the curious custom of domesticating canines and felines. To fulfill the prophecies of Isaiah 65:25 ("The wolf and the lamb shall feed together, and the lion shall eat straw like the bullock..."), we're just a step away if we prepare vegetarian food for our dogs and cats. There are companies specializing in such pet food; to purchase commercial pet food is to contract for the future murder of wild horses, cattle and dolphins—all victims of the current pet food industry. And just maybe your pets would like to dine with you, eating sufficient portions (or leftovers) of your natural, new diet.

Heal your life style and your family's diets. Alleviate the suffering of the planet and acknowledge the great advantages of the vegetarian way of life. Your personal "revolution" will make the next millennium a fantastic time to live in. Remember the statement of Victor Hugo: "There is no greater power than that of an idea whose time has come."

After many centuries of hypocrisy and the absurd, bloody murder of billions and billions of animals, the glorious VEGETARIAN TIME is rising! Mother Earth and all her dear living creatures need your distinguished contribution. Vegetarians are messengers of hope. Help history to write the first bloodless pages and heal itself. Your understanding will bless your brothers and sisters, showing the way out of dark habits where cruelty has dominated for far too long.

Be part of this network and meditate on the prophetic words of the famous Russian author Leo Tolstoy. More than one hundred years ago, he foresaw the coming of the Vegetarian Revolution and wrote:

> The wrongfulness, the immorality of eating animal food has been recognized by all mankind during all the conscious life of humanity. Why then have people generally not come to acknowledge this law? The answer is that the moral progress of humanity is always slow; but that the sign of true, not casual, progress is its uninterruptedness and its continual acceleration. And one cannot doubt that vegetarianism has been progressing in this manner.

So, dear friends, with open arms, open hearts and open minds, let's achieve that goal.

WE DON'T NEED TO KILL INNOCENT ANIMALS
TO BE WEALTHY, HEALTHY AND HAPPY.

The goal of the VEGETARIAN REVOLUTION is a superlative society with less crime, less disease, less violence and stress . . . an international, non-sectarian community of healthy and prosperous people ready to share with love the resources of the planet. If you are already a vegetarian, accept our deep gratitude. These pages can become in your hands an inexpensive and powerful tool to share and propagate your vision of how LIFE is suppose to be: one beautiful planet, one international community of brothers and sisters, one natural diet.

Envision an attractive, spiritual paradise where human beings are HUMANE again, totally free from the unavoidable bad reactions of killing for food. If you are not yet a vegetarian, we are here to reassure you. You will be glad to know that if you stop eating meat, you will immediately improve your life by gaining good physical and mental health.

This new diet will reward you with immediate economic, environmental, ethical, spiritual and nutritional benefits. Your purified consciousness will get a better understanding of your eternal spiritual nature, revealing a deeper insight into the hidden glorious dimensions we all have access to with a clear mind and a good heart. Good heart means generosity, love and peace. Enter a new and important chapter of your precious life. If you continue to eat death, you lose the wonderful opportunity to discover, enjoy and celebrate your own personal power. Sounds incredible? Or difficult to do? Fortunately, it is possible for all of us, and it has happened to many people before. The amazing energy of life is within everyone, rich or poor, ready to reveal the highest standard of our human potential.

Respect life and, miraculously, a marvelous karma-free prosperity will make you happy, healthy and wealthy. Understand that real wealth is not measured by how much money you have in the bank, but by how honest and sincere you are . . . and how rich and high you are on the ethical scale. Happiness happens when you enjoy life and serve with love—when you refrain from killing and instead are deeply concerned about the life of millions of humans struggling day after day just for mere survival. Invite yourself to this path of happiness, participate with any possible contribution to the feeding of families and children.   Plan to be actively part of the future reality, a self-sustaining vegetarian world. You have the extraordinary capacity to intensely awaken the conscience of many people around you. Don't feel discouraged by the pressure of political, financial and religious structures. All the major positive changes of history are started by small, happy and enthusiastic groups of people.

"One truth stands firm," said Nobel Peace Prize winner Albert Schweitzer, "all that happens in world history rests on something spiritual. If the spiritual is strong, it creates world history. If it is weak, it suffers world history." Another Nobel Peace Prize winner, Martin Luther King, Jr., stressed the importance of spirituality: "The means by which we live have outdistanced the ends for which we live. Our scientific power has outrun our spiritual power. We have guided missiles and misguided men."

"For the first time in history," warned Rachel Carson in *Silent Spring*, "every human being is now subjected to contact with dangerous chemicals, from the moment of conception until death." Even our battles against insects create collateral damage to our bodies, where insecticides show up, especially in the smaller constitutions of children. Yet there exist organic methods of agriculture that are gentle to the environment.

The privilege to be blissful and healthy is no concession to a cruel and senseless domination of the planet. Spirituality means sharing—caring for the welfare and happiness of all other forms of life. We are all one, whole ecological community. There is no way to escape this reality.

We deserve a better present, and the next generation a better future. And what is striking…please, let us repeat it once again: just by simply changing the food we put in our mouth, we can do the most to improve the quality of life for everyone living now on the planet. It could be so simple. John Robbins, author of *Diet for a New America* and President of the EarthSave Foundation, writes:

> In a world in which a child dies of starvation every two
> seconds, an agricultural system designed to feed our
> meat habit is a blasphemy. Thankfully, a rapidly grow-
> ing number of Americans are withdrawing support
> from this insane system by refusing to consume

animal flesh. For them, this new direction in diet-style is a way of joining hands with others and saying we will not support anymore a system which wastes such vast amounts of food while people in this world do not have enough to eat.

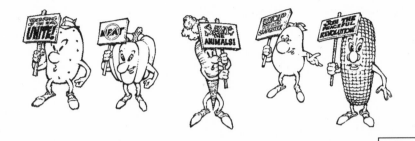

2

The Future Is Vegetarian

Food for 30 Billion People

What does the future hold? It is a simple and reasonable calculation as regards animal eating. In a few generations the world population will triple. The meat industry would be absolutely incapapble of tripling the production of meat. To do that, 11.1 billion acres of cropland and 22.5 billion acres of grazing are needed.

Guess what? This is more than the total area of the six inhabited continents! Cattle raising is already causing a shortage of groundwater, topsoil, forests and energy. So it is evident that it will be impossible to maintain the current levels of meat consumption per capita. So, why do we have to wait another century for the shift? The resources of this planet can easily provide a nutritious and tasty vegetarian diet for more than 30 billion people. The limit for a meat-centered diet is 8 billion. To survive, mankind will be forced to choose vegetarianism.

Vegetarian America

"People all over America will have very little choice but to become more vegetarian initially...and then totally vegetarian."
—Faith Popcorn, corporate trend-spotter

A People's Movement

"I didn't become a vegetarian for health reasons; I became vegetarian strictly for moral reasons. Vegetarianism will definitely become a people's movement."
—Dick Gregory, pacifist and civil rights leader

Simple Things To Do

"Have you tried your hand at edible gardening? Gardening is the number one recreational pursuit in America. You will be amazed at how much you can grow in even a tiny plot. Herbs, leafy greens, fruits and even corn can be grown quite handily in most urban settings."
—*50 Simple Things You Can Do To Save The Earth*, The Earthworks Press, Berkeley, California, USA

Victory Gardens

"During World War II, many Americans planted 'victory gardens.' These gardens supplied families with food at a crucial point in our national history. Though not in the midst of a world war, we still need victory gardens: this time, to combat the environmental crisis and regenerate the earth."
—*The Green Lifestyle Handbook,* Henry Holt & Company, New York

Twenty To One

Twenty vegetarians can be fed on the amount of land needed to feed one person consuming a meat-based diet.

Just Ten Percent

"Reducing meat production in the U.S. by just ten percent would release enough grain to feed sixty million people."
—Jean Mayer Harvard, nutritionist

Petroleum

The petroleum used in the United States would decrease by 60% if people adopted a vegetarian diet.

We Borrow It From Our Children

Number of acres of U.S. forest which have been cleared to create cropland, pasture land, and range land currently producing a meat-centered diet: 260,000,000

Number of acres of U.S. land which could be returned to forest if Americans adopted a meat-free diet and ceased exporting livestock feed: 204,000,000

Let's remember that "We don't inherit the land from our ancestors, we borrow it from our children."

The Time Will Come

"The food of the future will be fruit and grains. The time will come when meat will no longer be eaten. Medical science is only in its infancy, yet it has shown that our natural food is that which grows out of the ground."
—Abdu'l-Baha, founder of the Bahai Movement

Spirituality Will Defeat Meat Eating

In 1975, Alvin Toffler, author of *Future Shock* and *The Third Wave*, predicted, "I see a sudden rise of a religious movement in the West that restricts the eating of beef and thereby saves billions of tons of grain and provides a nourishing diet for the world as a whole." In the last twenty years, many spiritual groups and an international wave of new awareness has made, and is still making, millions of vegetarians all over the world.

Eliminating the Consumption of Meat

"Some sort of meeting of the minds is at work here. Those who have been vegetarian because they believe that not consuming animal product is morally or environmentally correct now have the support of a large body of scientific evidence suggesting that increasing the consumption of fruits, vegetables, grains and low fat dairy products, and decreasing or eliminating the consumption of meat, poultry and fish, may forestall the chronic ailments of aging like cancer and heart disease and can reverse the effects of atherosclerosis."
—*The New York Times*, July 8, 1992

My dear fellow humans, why wait another day? Make this vital decision the turning point of your life. Don't miss this opportunity. It is a winning decision in all respects. Nobody is going to lose.

If you are a leader, remember that we are in a democracy. One of the main functions of a good leader is to care for the well-being of the people, alerting society to the existence of any serious threat and thus deserving the people's support. Meat eating is a threat to the ecology, economy and spiritual progress of Earth. Develop a good strategy for dealing with this issue—help effect the transformation of meat eaters into vegetarians.

What is in jeopardy is the good health and the karma of America. Forty million Americans are obese, and more than 100 million are overweight. Statistics of heart disease and cancer are rising at a deadly rate each year. We are facing a major crisis, entirely created by misinformation on diet and life style. Homes, schools, temples and churches must recognize the urgency to create a new and happy American way of life. Wealth, technology and the learning system have been wasted, producing a pseudo-dream that along the way has lost the country's original values. America can be called the "Land of Liberty" only if there is liberty and justice for all living beings without violent discrimination. How long should it take to understand that animals are living beings?   I see, luckily, that the Vegetarian Revolution is happening throughout the world and is based on a new awareness that the most important power source for the next generations is a new kind of love and compassion. Of course, America will either be a successful leader in this new global vision or will become a dysfunctional, unhappy country full of sick and aggressive people.

Historically, in the West, vegetarianism started as a new culture around 1850. Great heroes of this health-oriented movement were the Reverend Sylvester Graham, the inventor of graham crackers; Ellen White, one of the founders of the Seventh Day Adventist Church; and Dr. John Harvey Kellogg, creator of the Kellogg breakfast cereals.

"The moral evils of a flesh diet are not less marked than are the physical ills. Flesh food is injurious to health and whatever affects the body has a corresponding effect on the mind and soul."
—Ellen G. White

"My refusing to eat flesh occasioned an inconvenience and I was frequently chided for my singularity."
—Ben Franklin

"I believe that every man who has ever been earnest to preserve his highest poetic faculties in the best condition has been particularly inclined to abstain from animal food."
—Henry David Thoreau

Vegetarian Advice from the Roman Empire

Read how clearly Plutarch, almost two thousand years ago, explains in his famous book *Moralia* that human beings were not anatomically created to eat flesh:

> We declare, then, that it is absurd for them to say that the practice of flesh-eating is based on Nature. For that man is not naturally carnivorous is, in the first place, obvious from the structure of his body. A man's frame is in no way similar to those creatures who were made for flesh eating: he has no hooked beak or sharp nails or jagged teeth, no strong stomach or warmth of vital fluids able to digest and assimilate a heavy diet of flesh. It is from this very fact, the evenness of our teeth, the smallness of our mouths, the softness of our tongues, our possession of vital fluids too inert to digest meat that Nature disavows our eating of flesh. If you declare that you are naturally designed for such diet, then first kill for yourself what you want to eat. Do it, however, only through your own resources, unaided by cleaver or cudgel or any kind of ax. Rather, just as wolves and bears and lions themselves slay what they eat, so you are to fell an ox with your own fangs or a boar with your jaws, or tear a lamb or hare in bits. Fall upon it and eat it still living, as animals do. But if you wait for what you eat to be dead, if you have qualms about enjoying the flesh while life is still present, why do you continue, contrary to nature to eat what possesses life? Even when it is lifeless and dead, however, no one eats the flesh just as it is; men boil it and roast it, altering it by fire and drugs, recasting and diverting and smothering with countless condiments the taste of gore so that the palate may be deceived and accept what is foreign to it.

We thank Harold Chermiss and William C. Helmbold, Harvard University Press, Cambridge, Massachusetts, for this superb translation of the ancient Latin text.

Diet for Outer Space

NASA is planning for space stations on the Moon and Mars. Besides the required budget and technology, the main problem is how to feed the astronauts. Frequent supply runs from our planet will not be easy or economically feasible. A conference at the Johnson Space Center in Houston assembled 40 experts to discuss the diet that looks sustainable in outer space. The clear answer was a vegetarian diet— and more specifically a vegan diet without any animal product. The space stations are "controlled ecological life support systems" and there is not enough space available to raise animals. Patricia Carey, EarthSave's executive director, said, "If we are gathered here because we know a vegan diet is the only diet that will work in a space station, why are we not applying that same knowledge to the space station planet Earth, that is also a controlled ecological life support system that currently works?"

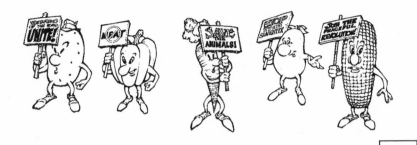

3

Animals Deserve
To Be Alive

Kill For Yourself The Animal You Want To Eat

"Let the advocate of animal food force himself to a decisive experiment on its fitness, and as Plutarch recommends, tear a living lamb with his teeth and, plunging his head into its vitals, slake his thirst with the steaming blood . . . then, and then only, would he be consistent."
—Percy Bysshe Shelley,
A Vindication of Natural Diet

Now I Can Look

"Now I can look at you in peace; I don't eat you anymore."
—Franz Kafka

Let Them Run

"If it runs away, don't eat it."
—Dr. Kellogg

Humane Animal Slaughter Is a Lie

"Many people nowadays have been lulled into a sense of compla-
cency by the thought that animals are now slaughtered 'humanely',
thus presumably removing any possible humanitarian objection to the
eating of meat. Unfortunately, nothing could be further from the actual
facts of life . . . and death. The entire life of a captive 'food animal'
is an unnatural one of artificial breeding, vicious castration and
hormone stimulation, feeding of an abnormal diet for fattening
purposes and, eventually, long rides in intense discomfort to the ultimate end. The holding pens, the electric prods and tail twisting, the
abject terror and fright, all these are still very much part of the most
'modern' animal raising, shipping, and slaughtering. To accept all this,
and only oppose the callous brutality of the last few seconds of the
animal's life, is to distort the word 'humane'."

> —*The Ethics of Vegetarianism*, an essay
> published by the North American Vegetarian
> Society

The Soul of Animals

"And God said, behold I have given you every plant yielding seed
which is on the face of all the earth and every tree yielding seed in its
fruit: you should have them as food. And to every beast of the earth,
and to every bird of the air, and to everything that creeps on the earth,
everything that has the breath of life, I have given every green plant
for food."

> —Genesis 1:29-30

The word animal comes from the Latin word *anima:* soul. This
evidence of eternal truth is again coming to light and the amount of
available information on animals and vegetarianism has really picked
up, even in the mainstream media. It is a blessing to see how many
people are reconsidering that all living creatures—"everything that has
the breath of life"—have a soul. It was the Greek philosopher Aristotle
who started the discrimination, establishing the anthropocentric idea

that only humans have rational souls. Thomas Aquinas later incorporated this idea into early Roman Christianity, even though it contradicts descriptions in the Bible that animals live in heaven.

To have recognition of a "soul" has been a long struggle, and not only for animals. For the first centuries of Christianity, some leading religious leaders denied that women have a soul. During the Synod of Macon (585), the Church leaders had the final debate whether or not women have souls. Up to the last century, black people and other races were heavily denied a "soul" by many ministers and scholars. In 1852, Josiah Priest wrote *Bible Defense of Slavery*. He and other authors claimed that blacks were subhuman—"Negroes are beasts and they have no souls to be saved." The Nazis, using the same principles, explained that the Jews were not "humans" and felt no regrets exterminating them. Animals, like innocent children, weak elders and peaceful women, have always been the victims of the cruel, sadistic behavior of authoritarian men.

The misconception that animals have no soul has misled many Christian leaders. Pope Pius XII stated that when animals are slaughtered or tortured in laboratories, humans shouldn't have emotional reactions: "Their cries should not arouse unreasonable compassion anymore than the red-hot metals undergoing the blows of the hammer." Recently, Pope John Paul II corrected that misunderstanding, proclaiming that "It is necessary and urgent that, following the example of the poor man (St. Francis), one decides to abandon any inconsiderate form of domination, capture and custody with respect to all creatures."

If we want to be part of a society that deserves to be called "civilized," we have to correct this gross mistake. Animals have a soul as we do and have the same absolute rights to enjoy life and express freely their feelings. They are not our slaves, but they can be good friends and wonderful companions.

In 1968, civil rights leader Dick Gregory compared the treatment of animals to the conditions of America's inner cities:

> Animals and humans suffer and die alike. If you had to kill your own hog before you ate it, most likely you would not be able to do it. To hear the hog scream, to see the blood spill, to see the baby being taken away

> from its momma, and to see the look of death in the
> animal's eye would turn your stomach. So you get the
> man at the packing house to do the killing for you.
>
> In like manner, if the wealthy aristocrats who are
> perpetrating conditions in the ghetto actually heard the
> screams of ghetto suffering, or saw the slow death of
> hungry little kids, or witnessed the strangulation of
> manhood and dignity, they could not continue the
> killing. But the wealthy are protected from such
> horror. If you can justify killing to eat meat, you can
> justify the conditions of the ghetto. I cannot justify
> either one.

The common truth is that we are all "souls" with a body. In this
life, we have a human body; others may have an animal body.

According to the Bible, animals have a soul. The exact Hebrew
term for animals in the Bible is *nephesh chaya*, which means, literally,
"living soul." The great German philosopher Schopenhauer criticized
how Christians treated animals:

> They are at once outlawed any philosophical morals;
> they are mere things, mere means to any ends whatso-
> ever. They can therefore be used for vivisection, hunt-
> ing, coursing, bullfights, and horse racing, and can be
> whipped to death as they struggle along with heavy
> carts of stone. Shame on such a morality that fails to
> recognize the eternal essence that exists in every living
> thing, and shines forth with inscrutable significance
> from all eyes that see the sun.

Unitarian minister Gary Kowalski wrote an entire book to prove
this logical truth, *The Souls of Animals.* "Animals," notes Kowalski,
"like us, are microcosms, they too care and have feelings; they too
dream and create; they too are adventuresome and curious about their
world. They too reflect the glory of the whole. Animals are living
souls. They are not things. They are not objects. They love. They
dance. They suffer. They know the peaks and chasms of being."

The following can be found in *The Science of Self-Realization*, published by The Bhaktivedanta Book Trust:

> Srila Prabhupada: Some people say, "We believe that animals have no soul." That is not correct. They believe animals have no soul because they want to eat the animals, but actually animals do have a soul.
>
> Reporter: How do you know that the animal has a soul?
>
> Srila Prabhupada: You can know, also. Here is the scientific proof. The animal is eating, you are eating; the animal is sleeping, you are sleeping; the animal is defending, you are defending; the animal is having sex, you are having sex; the animals have children, you have children; you have a living place, they have a living place. If the animal's body is cut, there is blood; if your body is cut, there is blood. So all these similarities are there. Now why do you deny this one similarity, the presence of the soul? That is not logical. You have studied logic? In logic there is something called analogy. Analogy means drawing a conclusion by finding many points of similarity. If there are so many points of similarity between human beings and animals, why deny one similarity? That is not logic. That is not science.

The Central Dilemma

"The researcher's central dilemma exists in an especially acute form of psychology: either the animal is not like us, in which case there is no reason for performing the experiment; or else the animal is like us, in which case we ought not to perform the experiment which would be considered outrageous if performed on one of us."

—Professor Peter Singer, author of
Animal Liberation

The Cause of the Protection of Animal Life

"Devoted as I was from boyhood to the cause of the protection of animal life, it is a special joy to me that the universal ethic of Reverence for Life shows that sympathy with animals, which is so often represented as sentimentality, to be a duty which no thinking man can escape."

—Dr. Albert Schweitzer (1875-1965)

Love the Animals

"You teach children about animals—piggies and lambs and cows and chickens—and then feed them these animals for lunch and supper."

—Candice Bergen, in an interview by *Parade* magazine

Lions and Wolves

"Can you really ask what reason Pythagoreans had for abstinence from flesh? For my part I rather wonder both by what accident and in what state of mind the first man touched his mouth to gore and brought his lips to the flesh of a dead creature, set forth tables of dead, stale bodies, and ventured to call food and nourishment the parts that had a little before bellowed and cried, moved and lived....It is certainly not lions or wolves that we eat out of self-defense; on the contrary, we ignore these and slaughter harmless, tame creatures without stings or teeth to harm us. Let them live for the duration of life they are entitled to by birth and being."

—Plutarch (46-119 C.E.), from *On Eating Flesh*

The Sacred Cow

"Perhaps the heaviest criticism of the pastoral culture of India is directed at the insistence of the farmers on protecting even sick and aged cows. Westerners find this to be the height of absurdity. At least THEY could be killed and eaten and sold. But no. Animal hospitals or nursing homes called goshallas, provided by government agencies or wealthy individuals in search of piety, offer shelter for old and infirm cows. This is thought to be a luxury that India cannot really afford, as these useless cows are seen to be but competitors for the already limited croplands and precious foodstuffs. The fact is, however, that India actually spends a great deal less on their aging cattle than Americans spend on their cats and dogs. And India's cattle population is six times that of the American pet population. The Indian farmer sees his cattle like dear members of the family. Since the farmers depend on the cattle for their own livelihood, it makes perfect sense both economically and emotionally to see to their well-being. In between harvests, the cattle are bathed and spruced up much like the average American polishes his automobile. Twice during the year, special festivals are held in honor of the cow. These rituals are similar to the American idea of Thanksgiving. Although in principle the same, there is a basic difference in the details of how we treat the turkey and how the more primitive Indians treat the cow. For India the cow represents the sacred principle of motherhood. She symbolizes charity and generosity because of the way she distributes her milk, which is essential for the nourishment of the young."

—Robin Winter, in *The Clarion Call* magazine

Hare Krishna Devi Dasi, a pioneer in restoring farm animals to their status as protected help-mates to mankind, writes about the origins of cow-killing economics:

> Lord Krishna says in the Bhagavad-gita that the activities of the productive society should be: agriculture, cow protection, and trade. As we drive down the road and see many prosperous hamburger chains, we may take for granted that cow slaughter has been a basic feature of civilizations outside India. But that is not the case. The ancient Egyptians prohibited cow slaughter. The Hebrews, among others, restricted it to religious sacrifices. Still today, the pastoral people of East Africa slaughter cows only during rituals and cere-

monies. And in modern communist China, even Mao Zedong himself observed, "Draft oxen are a treasure to the peasants."

Anthropologist Marvin Harris suggests that religious and ritual restrictions on cow slaughter and eating of cow flesh were not irrational laws but important tools for the welfare of society. The draft power or milk of the animal was too valuable to lose. In Europe in the late Middle Ages, the draft horse began to push the ox out of agriculture. In the 1700s, the Industrial Revolution speeded up cow slaughter. New farming machines and new crops such as clover and turnips made cows easier to raise for meat. And technological advances increased the output and efficiency of slaughterhouses. So producers could supply meat more cheaply. Factory life forced people to change what they ate. Unlike the farmer, the factory worker couldn't go home to a lunch of lentil stew or porridge. Bread and meat were more convenient. In *The Industrial Revolution* Frederick Dietz writes, "Since meat was coming to be more valuable than powers of draft in an ox, traditional breeds that provided milk and draft power tended to be replaced by new breeds of cattle." The Industrial Revolution bred beef cattle. In America until about 1840, when draft horses became more widespread, oxen were the main source of agricultural traction. A team of oxen could be bought for one sixth the price of a team of horses. Oxen could do the same work for less expense in feed, and oxen were resistant to disease.

Yet two factors made it possible and even profitable to raise cattle for slaughter. The first was the Native American crop maize—or corn—which gave much higher yields than European grains. The second was by taking land from the Native Americans, European immigrants could create much larger farms than in

Europe. The new American farmers were able to take hold of large plots of this fertile land, so with oxen the farmers could reap tons of grain more than they needed for their own subsistence. The farmers, of course, wanted to make money from the grain, but shipping it to the market was difficult. Roads were poor and carts were scarce. Smithsonian agricultural historian John Schlebecker relates the farmers unenlightened solution: "Corn-fed cattle and hogs which transported themselves provided one important way of moving the corn crop to market. The grain otherwise had to be transported by cart and wagon."

North American farmers also developed vital economic relations with the slave-powered sugar plantations of the West Indies. European plantation owners preferred to plant all their West Indian acreage in sugar, sell it at high prices, and import whatever else they needed for food. Corn, wheat, flour and bread from North America always found a ready market in the West Indies. The West Indians also bought large quantities of dried and salted meats. Thus, farming and cow killing began to assume an important place in American economic development.

The above is from "The Land, the Cows and Krishna" by Hare Krishna Devi Dasi, published in *Back to Godhead*, the magazine of the Hare Krishna Movement, January '92. You can contact her at The Ox Power Alternative Energy Club, 9B Stetson St., Brunswick, ME 04011.

Cows Can't Say No, But We Can

"Four multinational drug companies have invested more than half a billion dollars in the development and promotion of BGH. The battle over the approval and use of this hormone has significance for all areas of animal agriculture. If BGH gains acceptance, it will pave the way for the use of genetically engineered growth stimulants for pigs, sheep, and other farm animals. BGH itself has already been used in experiments to produce larger, faster growing chickens.

"Bovine Growth Hormone (BGH), also known as Bovine Somatotropin (BST), works by interfering with a cow's natural physiology. Lactation is artificially manipulated through hormone injections. Drug manufacturers claim that this will cause an increase of up to 20% in milk production. BGH is produced by extracting growth hormones from cows and using sophisticated gene-splicing techniques to create synthetic hormones. These hormones are then injected into dairy cows on a regular basis.

"BGH will also stimulate drug company profits by increasing the sales of other pharmaceuticals. As BGH forces cows to produce more milk than is healthy for their bodies, the cows become more susceptible to infection and disease. This, in turn, creates additional needs for antibiotics and other drugs—which these companies are all happy to provide."

> —from a special report *Turning Cows into High-Tech Milk Machines*, by the Humane Farming Association, Campaign Against Factory Farming, P.O. Box 3577, San Rafael, CA 94912.

Pain

"Pain is pain, whether it be inflicted on man or on beast."
—Dr. Humphrey Primatt

Do You Know That They Suffer?

"The question is not, can they reason? Nor, can they talk? But, can they suffer?"
—Jeremy Bentham

Be Kind To Beasts

"There is no religion without love, and people may talk as much as they like about their religion, but if it does not teach them to be kind to beasts as man, it is all a sham."
—Anna Sewell, author of *Black Beauty*

The Tyranny Of Humans

"The tyranny of humans over nonhumans is causing an amount of pain and suffering that can only be compared with that which resulted from the centuries of tyranny by white humans over black humans."
—Peter Singer, *Animal Liberation*

The True Parallel To Auschwitz

"…is there any credit balance for the battery hen, denied almost all natural functioning, all normal environment, lapsing steadily into deformity and disease, for the whole of her existence? It is in the battery shed and the broiler house, not in the wild, that we find the true parallel to Auschwitz. Auschwitz is a purely human invention."
—from a sermon of Austin Baker, Bishop of Salisbury, England (September 28, 1986)

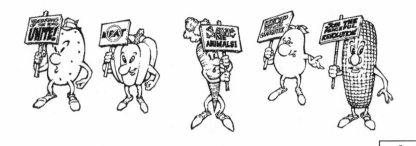

4

More Evidence

"The simple fact is that our diets have changed radically within the last 50 years, with great and often very harmful effects on our health. These dietary changes represent as great a threat to public health as smoking. In all, six of the ten leading causes of death in the United States have been linked to our diet."
—Senator George McGovern

Human anatomy and physiology are not similar to carnivorous animals. Human beings have stomach acid ten times less strong than meat-eating animals and their intestinal tract is six times their body length. The intestinal tract of meat-eating animals is only three times their body length, so decaying meat can pass out of the body quickly. The deteriorating health of many Americans is due to the dietary changes of the last fifty years, when meat became the main food. The National Academy of Sciences has recommended that people eat more fruits, vegetables and whole grains, decreasing the enormous consumption of meat. "Ischemic heart disease, cancer, diabetes and hypertension," wrote a Harvard professor in *Dietary Goals for the United States,* "are the diseases that kill us. They are epidemic in our population."

In addition to the fact that many honest doctors and scientists are proving, scientifically, that pieces of a dead body are not at all good for your health, we want to remind you of the hazardous risks of contracting diseases from the animals themselves. The horrible living conditions of all the poor animals raised for slaughter are not healthy. They suffer, crammed together in filthy, unclean, overcrowded confinements full of germs and viruses. These innocent creatures of God are reduced to consumable raw material. Their bodies, under the constant pressure of cruel treatment, become less resistant to diseases that they could have normally defeated. Fear, stress and pain release into the animal's system large quantities of adrenaline and other chemicals from the endocrine glands that are not healthy for the human body.

To protect the market value of animals, it is a common practice to give them antibiotics and large doses of hormones. Artificially their growth accelerates and their weight increases. Even after cooking, small parts of these chemicals are still active and enter the human body, accumulating and causing, after many years, devastating effects. Your body gets weak, wrinkled and deteriorates prematurely.

If federal standards were strictly respected, many slaughterhouses and butchers would soon go out of business. Some courageous animal rights groups are now revealing the criminal cover-up of various violations of the law by powerful meat industries. Meat is a huge business, and money often kept authorities and many scientists silent. It is a common belief that the U.S. Department of Agriculture protects the health of taxpayers through meat inspection. The reality is that only one out of every quarter million slaughtered animals is tested for toxic chemical residues. Now, some honest researchers working inside this corrupt system are coming out with startling evidence: besides the many dangerous diseases commonly found in animal flesh, they have discovered rodent feces, cockroaches, rust and many germs harmful to the human body.

Several well-organized studies have scientifically shown that in the last thirty years— after tobacco and alcohol—the consumption of meat is the greatest single cause of mortality in Western Europe, the United States, Australia and other affluent areas of the world. This conclusion was also present in the report *Dietary Goals for the United States*, printed by the Senate Select Committee on Human Needs in 1977.

Meat eaters eat more cholesterol than the body needs. *The Journal of the Norwegian Medical Association* (in the article "What is the Experts' Opinion on Diet and Coronary Heart Diseases?") points out that when a human accumulates excess cholesterol on the inner walls of the arteries, it constricts the flow of blood to the heart and can kill the person by causing strokes, heart diseases and high blood pressure disorders. The agreement about the link between meat and heart diseases came from the results of research done by more than 200 scientists from different parts of the world.

"Another problem," wrote Sara Shannon in *Diet for The Atomic Age*, "is that meat is high on the food chain and can contain a high concentration of radioactive contaminants. An interesting point is that, unlike ours, the intestinal tracts of carnivorous animals are relatively short, so that they can quickly process meat without absorbing toxic substances. In contrast, it takes anywhere from several hours to over one day for meat, which is very low in fiber, to go through the human intestinal tract. During this time, it decays and putrefies, so we can't properly digest and assimilate the useful nutrients it originally contained. Instead, toxic by-products are left in the body to clutter the bloodstream and lower our health. The slow intestinal transit time also can contribute to increased internal radiation absorption. So it is not surprising that there is a high correlation between meat intake and colon cancer. In addition to the hazards posed by all the various levels of contamination, the cooking of meat can also lead to health problems. Cancer-causing and mutation-causing substances are formed during broiling, roasting and barbecuing."

A high-fiber diet is an excellent preventive medicine. Fiber cannot be absorbed or digested and is needed by the intestines to move their contents through the digestive tract, preventing and relieving constipation. Fiber promotes the growth in the intestines of beneficial bacteria, synthesizes B vitamins, produces enzymes that improve digestion, and prevents harmful microorganisms from multiplying and producing toxins or carcinogens. This has a detoxifying effect and reduces stress on the immune system.

Where to find fiber? In whole foods—whole grains like barley, rice, kasha, millet and wheat berries; legumes such as peas, soybeans, blackbeans, lentils, and lima beans; and in fresh fruits and vegetables. Whole grains actually have more fiber than fruits and vegetables.

High Fiber = Low Fat

"Cancer of the colon, prostate, and breast, and other disorders, such as diverticulitis, appendicitis, hemorrhoids, and varicose veins, are all related to a high-fat diet. A diet high in fiber will be low in fat. Those who switch to a high-fiber diet lose weight, keep cholesterol levels down, and need no laxatives."
> —Leslie Cerier, personal fitness counselor, in *The Little Book of Secrets*, Martin Edelston, Publisher

Cholesterol

Eggs contain one of the densest concentrations of cholesterol available. When people eat eggs, cholesterol pours through the bloodstream, increasing the risk of heart disease. The human body makes all the cholesterol it needs and when extra cholesterol is eaten, only 100 mg. a day can be eliminated. The rest begins clogging the arteries.

Good Heart

"Ninety to ninety-seven percent of heart disease can be prevented by a vegetarian diet."
> —*Journal of the American Medical Association*

Coronary Death

Coronary Death Rate: Total Vegetarian (14%), Lacto-ovo-vegetarian (39%), Non-vegetarian (56%)
> —Keith Akers, *A Vegetarian Sourcebook*

Stop Cancer

"I have found of twenty-five nations largely eating flesh, nineteen had a high cancer rate and only one had a low rate, and that of thirty-five nations eating little or no flesh, none had a high rate."

> —Rollo Russell, in his Notes on the Causation of Cancer, published in *Cancer and Other Diseases from Meat Consumption* and reported by Blanche Leonardo, Ph.D.

"People may be able to prevent many common types of cancer by eating less fatty meats and more vegetables and grains."

> —from a Report of the American Academy of Sciences, *Diet, Nutrition and Cancer*, published by the National Academy Press, Washington.

Vegetables Defeat Cancer

"Vitamin C and E and certain chemicals called indoles, found in cabbage, Brussels sprouts, and related vegetables in the crucifer family, are potent and safe inhibitors of certain carcinogens."

> —from a report of the Massachusetts Institute of Technology

Eat More Vegetables

"People may be able to prevent many common types of cancer by eating less fatty meats and more vegetables and grains."

> —from a Report of the American Academy of Sciences, *Diet, Nutrition and Cancer*, published by the National Academy Press, Washington.

Prevention

"People living in the areas with a high recorded incidence of carcinoma of the colon tend to live on diets containing large amounts of fat and animal protein; whereas those who live in areas with a low incidence live on largely vegetarian diets with little fat or animal matter."

> —from the medical magazine *Lancet*

Cancer Can Be Prevented

The Cure for All Cancers is the astounding title of a book written by Hulda Clark, Ph.D., N.D. In 1990, Dr. Clark discovered a certain parasite, for which she found evidence in every cancer, regardless of type. She set a goal of 100 cases to be cured of cancer before publishing her findings; that mark was passed in December 1992. This important book seems to have saved the lives of many people, and may help save you or someone you know.

She doesn't suggest a treatment for cancer but a cure for removing the parasite known as human intestinal fluke. She writes:

> You are always picking up parasites! Parasites are everywhere around you! You get them from other people, your family, yourself, your home, your pets and undercooked meat! I believe the main source of the intestinal fluke is undercooked meat. After we are infected with it in this way, we can give it to each other through blood, saliva, semen, and breast milk, which means kissing on the mouth, sex, nursing, and childbearing.

Meat could be the source. Are we getting metacercaria from eating animals that have the parasite? The animal's blood has eggs, miracidia, redia, cercaria and metacercaria in it. We swallow all those live eggs.

The metacercaria are meant to attach themselves to our intestine and grow larger, into adults that lay more eggs, which in turn hatch into more miracidia. Propyl alcohol (a commonly-used by-product of the petrochemical industry, present in most cleaning agents) promotes this parasite's development in the liver as well other tissues that have toxins in them. This causes a population explosion and ortho-phosphotyrosine production, namely CANCER. This raises the possibility—in fact, the probability—that our meat animals are the "biological reservoir," the source of infection, of the cancer-causing parasite!

The best cancer prevention choice is to BECOME A PURE VEGETARIAN IMMEDIATELY!

The Healing Food

"It is a true statement: An apple a day keeps the doctor away. Apples lower cholesterol and blood pressure, stabilize blood sugar, block cancer, and kill infectious viruses. Bananas prevent and heal ulcers, lower cholesterol and keep your heart beating regularly. Carrots cut the risk of lung cancer, reduce the blood fats that cause heart attacks and strokes, and help prevent colon cancer. Blueberries prevent damage to blood vessels. Cherries prevent cavities. Grapes fight tooth decay. Olive oil fights cancer, heart disease and aging. Cabbage prevents ulcers. Whole grain breads recharge your energy levels and fight colon cancer."

> —Dr. Julian Whitaker, *Forbidden Cures*

Don't Tell the Doctor You Are Vegetarian

"I recommend to everyone who is vegetarian never to tell his doctor, because doctors cannot stand vegetarians. In the Religion of Modern Medicine, doctors believe in red meat, and if you tell a doctor that you are a vegetarian, he will curse you. He will say to you: 'You are going to develop vitamin B12 deficiency,' and he will threaten you in other ways as well. So as far as I am concerned, you should never confess to the doctor that you are vegetarian. The doctor is an important political figure with enormous influence, both personally and through his organizations on legislative and judicial activity. Therefore, his high tolerance for environmental pollution and pollution of the food supply is leading to a national catastrophe."

> —from an interview of Robert S. Mendelsohn,
> M.D., author of *Confessions of a Medical
> Heretic*, published in *The Clarion Call*, a
> theistic alternative magazine for the modern
> age

Eat the Poison

"The animals are kept alive and fattened by continuous administration of tranquilizers, hormones, antibiotics and 2,700 other drugs.

The process starts even before birth and continues long after death. Although these drugs will still be present in the meat when you eat it, the law does not require that they be listed on the package."
— Gary and Steven Null, *Poisons in Your Body*, Arco Press

Healthy and Vegetarian

"The central question about vegetarian diet used to be whether it was healthy to eliminate meat and other animal foods. Now, however, the main question has become whether it is healthier to be vegetarian than to be a meat eater. The answer to both questions, based on currently available evidence, seems to be yes."
— Jane E. Brody, New York Times News Service

Pure Food

"Our modern diet is a nutritional disaster. Our grains are first devitalized by grinding away most of their vitamins and minerals; then they are liberally laced with unbalanced proportions of sugar, salt, and various additives. Convenience foods are for the convenience of the food industry. Packaged food is refined and preserved with additives so that it can be shipped great distances and stored on grocery shelves without spoiling. Some food additives have been shown to cause cancer in rats. Almost three thousand chemicals are approved for use in our daily food supply; the average American consumes up to nine pounds yearly of these additives."
— Doctor Michael Lesser, *Nutrition and Vitamin Therapy*

The purity of our daily food is very important for the maintenance of our health. The dye used for many years by the U.S. Department of Agriculture to stamp meats "Choice", "Prime", or "U.S. No. 1"— Violet Dye No. 1—has now been banned as a probable carcinogen. Who will pay for the damage that has been caused to many uninformed citizens?

Even if it takes time and a little more money to go "organic," consider the long-term effects of "junk food", falsely advertised as good, tasty, healthy and convenient.

Always prefer fresh, untreated, and unprocessed foods. Processed foods can make you sick. There are no rules on the amount of salt that can be used in food processing. The human kidneys can handle no more then 10 grams of mineral salts a day, and the average American diet consumes daily 20 to 25 grams of salt. These salts are not eliminated and are stored in various parts of the body, causing obesity, high blood pressure, kidney and heart disease, arthritis and rheumatism.

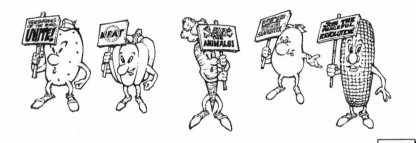

5

Proteins and Vitamins

Protein Power

From *The Vegetarian Guide,* printed by The San Francisco Vegetarian Society:

Q. Is it necessary to combine plant foods to make a complete protein?
A. No, combining plant foods such as rice and beans at the same meal is unnecessary. Protein is made up of amino acids. The essential amino acids are the 8 out of 20 amino acids that must be supplied in the diet because our bodies cannot make them. Protein combining in order to get all of the essential amino acids during the same meal is actually a myth propagated by Frances M. Lappe´ in her book *Diet For a Small Planet.* In the revised edition, Lappe´ writes:

> *Diet For a Small Planet* helped create a new myth, that to get the protein you need without meat you have to conscientiously combine non-meat sources to create a protein that is as usable by the body as meat protein. Protein complementary is not the myth; it works. The myth is that complementing proteins is necessary for most people on a low or non-meat diet. With a healthy

and varied diet, concern about protein complementarity is not necessary for most of us.

One of the foremost authorities on nutrition, the American Dietetic Association, stated that "A plant-based diet provides adequate amounts of all amino acids if a variety of foods are eaten over the course of the day." This means that protein combining, such as eating beans and rice at each meal to form a "complete" protein, is unnecessary as long as both are eaten at some time during the day.

Three essential amino acids occurring in especially lower amounts in plant foods are tryptophan, lysine and methionine. Foods which are good sources of these three essential amino acids are listed below.

TRYPTOPHAN: peanuts, peas, cashews and seeds.

LYSINE: brewers' yeast, wheat germ, beans and seitan (high protein wheat flour, also called gluten).

METHIONINE: whole soybeans and soy flour, whole grains, sesame and pumpkin seeds.

Q. Do vegetarians get enough vitamins and minerals?
A. Even vegans can obtain necessary nutrients by eating a well-balanced diet. Otherwise, nutritional deficiencies are most likely to occur for the vitamins D, B12 and riboflavin, and the minerals, iron, calcium and zinc.

To avoid deficiencies, include these foods in the diet: whole grains, legumes (beans, tofu, peas), nuts (almonds), seeds (pumpkins and sesame), dried fruit, mushrooms, cabbage, beets, yellow and green leafy vegetables (squash and broccoli).

It is important to note that absorption of iron from grains and legumes is increased by including a good source of Vitamin C at that meal. Also calcium is best absorbed when sesame seeds are hulled, in the form of sesame butter (tahini) or at least very well chewed.

Vitamins D and B12 require a bit more planning to be included in the diet. Vitamin D is made by our bodies when sunlight hits the skin. Soy milk may be fortified with Vitamin D. Vitamin B12 may be found in small amounts in tempeh (fermented soy product), spirulina and seaweed. Some cereals (Grape-Nuts brand) are fortified with Vitamin

B12. Nutritional yeast (available in health food stores) often contains plenty of Vitamin B12.

If the above mentioned foods are not eaten regularly in the diet, vegetarians may consider taking supplements to avoid nutritional deficiency diseases.

Q. Do vegetarians get enough protein in their diets?
A. Vegetarians can get plenty of protein from plant foods they eat: grains, vegetables, nuts and fruits. The U.S. Recommended Dietary Allowance (revised in 1989) for protein is:

> Females: weight 128 lb., age 19-24, protein 46 grams
> weight 138 lb., age 25-50, protein 50 grams

> Males: weight 160 lb., age 19-24, protein 58 grams
> weight 174 lb., age 25-50, protein 63 grams

However, the World Health Organization (WHO) maintains that less protein is necessary—only 37 grams for the average man and 29 grams for the average woman.

The Protein Myth

"The official daily recommendation for protein has gone down from the 150 grams recommended twenty years ago to only 45 grams today. Why? Because reliable worldwide research has shown that we do not need so much protein, that the actual daily need is only 30 to 45 grams. Protein consumed in excess of the actual daily need is not only wasted, but actually causes serious harm to the body and is even causatively related to such killer diseases as cancer and heart disease. In order to obtain 45 grams of protein a day from your diet, you don't have to eat meat; you can get it from a 100 percent vegetarian diet of a variety of grains, lentils, nuts, vegetables and fruits."
　　　　　—Dr. Paavo Airola, *Vegetarian Times*, August '82

"Actually, it's nearly impossible not to get enough protein, no matter what you eat, as long as you eat enough calories. The misunderstanding of human protein requirements started in the early part of this century, when two scientists published the results of a study showing that rats fed vegetable proteins grew more slowly than rats fed animal proteins. We now know that humans and rats have very different protein requirements and that people can get all the protein they need from plant sources. A bigger problem is the excess protein in most Americans' diet, which is implicated in osteoporosis, kidney failure, colon cancer, and other health problems."

—Neal D. Barnard, M.D., *The PETA Guide to Compassionate Living*

Where Are The Amino Acids?

"Plants can synthesize amino acids from air, earth and water, but animals are dependent on plants for protein, either directly by eating plants or indirectly by eating an animal which has eaten and metabolized plants. Only the vegetable kingdom is capable of producing protein. Thus, humans have the option of obtaining it directly and with great efficiency from plants or indirectly and at great expense, both financially and in terms of resources consumed, from animal flesh. There are thus no amino acids in flesh that animals do not derive from plants, or that humans cannot also derive from plants. Moreover, eating foods from the plant kingdom has the added advantage of combining amino acids with other substances that are essential to the proper utilization of protein: carbohydrates, vitamins, minerals, enzymes, hormones, chlorophyll, and other elements that only plants can supply."

—Steven Rosen, *Diet for Transcendence*

The Vegetarian Food Pyramid

I suggest this daily guide to food choices:

SPARINGLY: fats, oils and sweets. These foods provide calories and are low in nutrients. Use visible fats sparingly. Limit desserts to two or three per week. Limit food high in salt.

MODERATELY: legumes, beans, nuts, seeds and meat alternatives, 2-3 servings. Low-fat or non-fat milk, yogurt, fresh cheese, and/or fortified alternatives, like soy or tofu milk, 2-3 servings.

GENEROUSLY: fruits, fresh and dried, 2-4 servings. Vegetables, 3-5 servings.

LIBERALLY: whole grains, breads, cereals, and pasta, 6-11 servings.

Water

We are made of water. More then 90% of the blood is composed of water. Water makes up 71% of our body weight; 75% of our muscles, 90% of our brain, 69% of our liver and 22% of our bones are just water.

Oxygen and water are the substances we need the most. Pollution is threatening the quality of these two vital sources of energy. An important function of good water is the flushing out of toxins and excess salts from the body. Tap water is full of chemicals which attack the arteries, veins and vital organs. Bottled water is not completely pure.

Patrick and Gael Crystal Flanagan's book, *Elixir of the Ageless, You Are What You Drink* (Vortex Press, 22 S. San Francisco St., Suite 219, Flagstaff, AZ 86001), helps us understand how important pure water is for our health. They write:

> The very best way of cleansing the impurities from the body is through the use of high zeta potential liquid crystal colloids. The second best way of completely cleansing the human body and nourishing the cells is by drinking large quantities of pure mineral-free distilled water.

Dr. Flanagan continued the research of Dr. Coanda, the father of Fluid Dynamics. Coanda traveled to remote mountain valleys where people lived over 100 years, maintaining youthful health. He visited the Hunzaland in the Karakorum Mountains of Tibet, the Vilcabamba of Ecuador and the Georgians in the former Soviet Union. He discovered that water, the special cloudy colloidal water, was the main cause of their centenarian healthy life. After 24 years of research, Dr. Flanagan claims that he found the way to recreate the same water of the Hunza.

"In fact today, colloids may be regarded as important, perhaps the most important connecting link between the organic and the inorganic world."
—Wolfgang Pauli

I suggest fasting regularly, using only distilled water; however, if you feel inspired by the amazing power of the colloid water, learn more about the importance of colloids in the living system.

A good and pure blood system is the real key to health and longevity. A pure vegetarian diet and good water can eliminate easily the cellular waste and all the toxins. Meat eating introduces in the blood poisons, bacteria, hormones, disease, viruses and the leftover medicines and antibiotics given to the animals.

The Nobel Prize in Medicine was given to Dr. Alexis Carrel when he proved theoretically that the life of the cell is unlimited if it is fed properly and all the toxic waste removed. A balanced vegetarian diet can protect and defend the cells of your body, preventing diseases and deterioration.

Eight Glasses A Day Keep Fat Away

Incredible as it may seem, water is the single most important catalyst in losing weight and keeping it off. Although most of us take it for granted, water may be the only true "magic potion" for permanent weight loss. From the *Snowbird Diet*, by Donald S. Robertson, M.D. and Carol P. Robertsch, Warner Books:

> Studies have shown that a decrease in water intake will cause fat deposits to increase, while an increase in water intake can actually reduce fat deposits. The kidneys can't function properly without enough water. When they don't work to capacity, some of their load is dumped onto the liver. One of the liver's primary functions is to metabolize stored fat into usable energy

for the body. But, if the liver has to do some of the kidney's work, it can't operate at full throttle. As a result, it metabolizes less fat, more fat remains stored in the body and weight loss stops. When the body gets less water, it perceives this as a threat to survival and begins to hold on to every drop. Water is stored in extracellular spaces (outside the cells). This shows up as swollen feet, legs and hands. The best way to overcome the problem of water retention is to give your body what it needs—plenty of water. Only then will stored water be released. If you have a constant problem with water retention, excess salt may be to blame. Your body will tolerate sodium only in a certain concentration. The more salt you eat, the more water your system retains to dilute it. But getting rid of unneeded salt is easy—just drink more water. As it's forced through the kidneys, it takes away excess sodium.

Water helps to maintain proper muscle tone by giving muscles their natural ability to contract and by preventing dehydration. It also helps to prevent the sagging skin that usually follows weight loss—shrinking cells are buoyed by water, which plumps the skin and leaves it clear, healthy and resilient.

During weight loss, the body has a lot more waste to get rid of—all that metabolized fat must be shed. Again, adequate water helps flush out the waste.

When the body gets too little water, it siphons what it needs from internal sources. The colon is one primary source. Result? Constipation. But when a person drinks enough water, normal bowel function usually returns.

On the average, a person should drink eight 8-ounce glasses every day. That's about 2 quarts. Cold water is absorbed into the system more quickly than warm water. And some evidence suggests that drinking cold water can actually help to burn calories.

To utilize water most efficiently during weight loss, follow this schedule:

MORNING: 1 quart consumed over a 30-minute period

NOON: 1 quart consumed over a 30-minute period

EVENING: 1 quart consumed between five and six o' clock

When the body gets the water it needs to function optimally, its fluids are perfectly balanced. When this happens, you have reached the "breakthrough point". What does this mean?

Endocrine-gland function improves. Fluid retention is alleviated as stored water is lost. More fat is used as fuel because the liver is free to metabolize stored fat. Natural thirst returns. There is a loss of hunger almost overnight.

Water Use

In California, the number of gallons of water needed to produce 1 edible pound of: tomatoes (23), lettuce (23), potatoes (24), wheat (25), carrots (33), apples (49), oranges (65), grapes (70), milk (130), eggs (544), chicken (815), pork (1630), beef (5214). It takes one year for a person to use 5200 gallons of water showering (at 5 showers a week, 5 minutes per shower, with a rate of 4 gallons per minute).

Warning About Milk

We accept the idea that pure milk could be part of your vegetarian diet, but we do not guarantee the quality of milk you buy in the market. It is often full of hormones and antibiotics. At least half the 10 million dairy cows in the U.S. spend their lives in crowded, concrete-floored milking pens or barns, artificially inseminated on what factory farmers call the "rape rack". The dairy cow's male calves are sold to the veal industry within two days. If you want to drink milk, support those groups and communities that are not killing cows. For more information contact The International Society for Cow Protection, ISCOWP Office, RD 1 NBU #28, Moundsville, WV 26041, tel (304) 843-1270.

Herbs, Vitamins and Supplements

We suggest the reading of the *Vitamin Bible* by Earl Mindell, a scientific research that can guide you in the complex world of vitamins and nutritional supplements. It is proven that the intelligent and correct use of supplements can prevent you from many diseases. The market in the last few years has "exploded" and one can find hundreds of different brands promising miraculous benefits. Choosing supplements, you need to consult an expert, at least in the beginning; don't blindly accept the promises of labels. We suggest avoiding the use of synthetic vitamins. A quick example, synthetic vitamin C contains only ascorbic acid. Natural C from rose hips contains bioflavonoids, the entire C complex, which make Vitamin C much more effective. According to allergist Dr. Theron Randolph, "A synthetically derived substance may cause a reaction in a chemically susceptible person when the same material of natural origin is tolerated, despite the two substances having identical chemical structure."

In his book *Young Again*, Dr. Julian Whitaker deplores the fact that doctors don't tell their patients: "Vitamins can save your life!" He says that is almost criminal. If this news were to be broadcast widely, hundreds of thousands of people can easily save their lives. "Scientists have isolated the chemicals that cause most of the health problems you get as you age," explains Dr. Whitaker. "They are called oxygen-free radicals, and they attack every cell in your body, causing them to age. They attack your arteries and make them clog up faster, and they can make healthy cells cancerous. Scientists found that certain vitamins round up oxygen-free radicals and throw them out of your body before they can harm you!"

A six-year Harvard study of 21,000 doctors showed that those who took regular beta-carotene (vitamin A) supplements had half as many strokes, heart attacks and other heart problems as those who did not! In another Harvard study, nurses who took Vitamin E had 36% less risk of heart attack than those who didn't. A UCLA study of 11,348 adults showed that death rates are 45% lower in men with high levels of Vitamin C in their diets. And men who took regular Vitamin C supplements lived five years longer than those who didn't. Researchers were also surprised to discover that people who eat food grown in selenium-rich soil have the lowest cancer rates.

Good vegetarian nutrition and pure natural supplements can maximize your health and longevity. Drug companies are not completely innocent. They have this information but want you to believe that toxic drugs, painful tests and dangerous surgeries are your best medicine. Nature is filled with powerful remedies that could maintain your body in good shape.

Dr. Whitaker warns against arrogant doctors, knife-happy surgeons and greedy drug companies: "Drug companies bribe doctors to push their drugs! Doctors get free vacations, cellular phones, even free education for prescribing certain drugs, whether or not they are good for you."

Hippocrates, called the Father of Medicine, and the ancient Ayurvedic medical science of India left the same message: Food should be your best medicine. The kitchen should become the healing center of your home. "Epidemiological evidence," wrote Dr. H. Kesteloot, "overwhelmingly points toward nutrition as the major determinant of life expectancy."

Scientists and doctors should make an honest commitment to educate people that vegetarianism is a very powerful preventive measure that can save people's lives. The best and cheapest health plan comes from the vegetarian diet.

Vitamin Issues: Vitamin Supplements Can Cut Billions In Health Care Costs

The U.S. health care system could save $ 8.7 billion annually from reduced hospitalization that result from five major diseases, if Americans consumed optimal levels of the antioxidant vitamins C, E and beta-carotene. The $ 8.7 billion figure implies a five-year savings of more than $43.5 billion.

These numbers are part of an economic analysis, released September 22, 1993, at the Council for Responsible Nutrition's 20th anniversary annual conference in Washington D.C. The study by Pracon, Inc., a Virginia-based economic analysis firm, concluded that these figures represent only one portion of the potential savings, since hospitalizations represent only a piece of the total medical costs of the diseases studied, according to Steven Pashko, Ph.D., Pracon senior director and project leader on the study.

For more information, call (202) 872-1488 or fax (202) 872-9594.

Phytoestrogens Can Help You

Researchers have found that phytoestrogens may play a role in health maintenance and disease prevention, much like the antioxidants.

A study of the American Dietetic Association shows that beans, sprouts, tofu and soy drinks contain a substantial amount of phytoestrogens. When ingested they may act like hormones. Researchers are checking out that phytoestrogens may have an anti-estrogen effect in premenopausal women, which could mean a decrease in the risk of breast cancer. On the other hand, for postmenopausal women who have 60% less estrogen produced by the body, phytoestrogens may have an estrogen effect that may reduce menopausal symptoms. Low estrogen levels after menopause are linked to a higher incidence of osteoporosis and increased risk of cardiovascular disease in women.

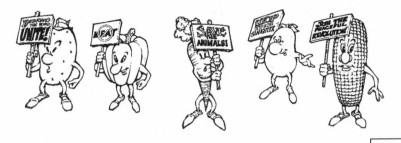

6

Vegetarians Live Longer

Populations eating a lot of meat (Eskimos, Greenlanders and Siberian tribes) live very short lives; the average life span is little more than 30 years. Other groups living in the same harsh climate live much longer if they eat less or no meat at all. It is scientifically proven that vegetarians live longer. Now, many scientists say that 120 years is probably the "design life" of the human body. Deaths today are premature. The main causes of death today are:

1) Heart Disease
2) Cancer
3) Stroke
4) Accidents
5) Chronic lung disease
6) Pneumonia and influenza
7) Diabetes
8) Suicide
9) Liver disease
10) Atherosclerosis

Six of the leading causes of death have been linked to diet.

According to the Center for Disease Control and Prevention, this is what determines good health:

*Life style (53%)
*Environment (19%)
*Heredity (18%)
*Medical care (10%).

The paradox is that medical care is the smallest contributor to health, but in the last 25 years healthcare spending has risen 25 times. Life style choices are the predominant factor. Eighty percent of all disease has been linked to only five factors, all related to life style choice: poor diet, smoking, alcohol, obesity, and unsafe sex. Americans tend to eat without knowing the correlation between what they put in their mouths and a wide range of degenerative diseases.

The constant advertising of fast food through the media is only increasing the problem. Studies confirm that vegetarians tend to be thinner and live longer. Many of these studies show the vegetarian diet to be lower in saturated fats and cholesterol.

The real key to having a better and healthier life is an intelligent plan of prevention. However, prevention is not taken very seriously by hospitals and government agencies. The same government that pays millions of dollars on studies to show pork and beef can add to health problems serves the very same meats in the schools to the most precious of our resources—our children. Hospitals, where the physicians may eat a vegetarian diet themselves, serve roast beef and white bread to their patients—the very ones who need the healthiest diet.

Many people are starting to take personal charge of their health, adjusting bad living patterns and exploring alternative medicine. The "holistic" approach—one that considers the individual a harmonious combination of body, mind and spirit—is getting the attention of 1/3 of all Americans. This portion of the population is paying, out of its own pocket, almost $15 billion a year for these unconventional therapies. The praticioners of alternative medicine are often doctors who are dissatisfied with the standard system.

America is the richest country in the world but ranks only seventeenth in life expectancy.

Thousands of years ago, the great prophet Isaiah foresaw a new world:

> For behold, I create new heavens and a new earth,
> Former things shall no more be remembered nor shall
> they be called to mind.
> Rejoice and be filled with delight,
> you boundless realms which I create;
> There no child shall ever again die an infant,
> no old man fail to live out his life:
> every boy shall live his hundred years before he dies.

His ancient insight about the future of mankind was completely vegetarian, a whole new perspective of relationships with one another will bless this planet with true everlasting peace:

> Then the wolf shall live with the sheep, and the leopard lie down with the kid;
> The calf and the young lion shall grow up together,
> and a little child shall lead them;
> The cow and the bear shall be friends, and their
> young shall lie down together.
> The lion shall eat straw like cattle; the infant shall
> play over the hole of the cobra, and the young child
> dance over the viper's nest.
> Men shall build houses and live to inhabit them,
> plant vineyards and eat their fruit.

These lines speak for themselves—the plea is a call for universal and eternal peace. Isaiah goes beyond denouncing animal sacrifices and offers an inspiring and poetic vision of the Kingdom of God. The race of human beings was created vegetarian and found itself in a position where it must either eat flesh or perish. Some of the gentle humans, who had lived happily in the Garden of Eden for so many years, eating the fruits and seeds which God had given them, started to kill and eat the flesh of their fellow creatures. Now the time has come to go back to the diet given by God himself in Genesis: "I give all plants that bear seed everywhere on earth, and every tree bearing fruit which yields seed: they shall be your food."

Longevity

I have been in India and had the great fortune to meet some powerful yogis, some of them centenarians. Not one was a meat eater; they are all vegetarians. At the Khumba Mela in Allahabad, in 1989, I met Devraha Baba, universally known in India as a great healer and spiritual guide. Many reliable sources confirmed that he was two hundred years old. In 1893, Swami Vivekananda met him before coming to the World Parliament of Religions in Chicago. At that time he was already "old" and famous. When I asked him what to eat, he told me *sattvic* food.

Sattva means truth and goodness; this is how yogis define vegetarian food. Explains Bhaktivedanta Swami Prabhupada:

> The Bhagavad-gita describes three categories of food. Sattvic food such as fruits, vegetables, cereals, pulses, nuts, milk, butter etc. promote longevity, intellect and strength, while granting pleasure, peace of mind, compassion, non-violence and equanimity, and save the body, heart and mind from all impurities. Rajasic food includes very hot, sour, bitter, spicy and dry substances and creates sorrow, disease and tensions. Tamasic food, like meat, lead men to evil deeds, cloud their intellect and give rise to diseases and other evil qualities.

When I asked Devraha Baba about his own diet, one of his disciples answered, smiling, that after a long life as a strict vegetarian, he didn't eat anymore. He relied on sunlight, pure water of the Holy River Ganges and clean air.

In New Delhi that same year, I met one of the most prominent Ayurvedic doctors of India, Bhagavan das. He has written many books on the subjects of food, healing and yoga and studied personally the life and eating habits of many yogis. He explained that yogis are all strictly vegetarian; and some are even capable of fasting for months, sustaining themselves through the mystical absorption of *prana* and the invisible subtle elements of food. They just eat vibrations, pure energy. Modern science understands more and more that the entire cosmic manifestation—on every plane, in every form, at all times—is energy. This vital energy—called *prana* in India, *chi* in Chinese, *mana* among Polynesian healers—sustains and perpetuates this visible universe. Recently this vitalizing force has been called bioplasma by Russian researchers and orgone energy by the German scientist Wilhelm Reich.

Albert Einstein, a vegetarian and considered one of the greatest geniuses of all times, said, "The knowledge about that which we know is only a fraction of that which we do not know..."

The variety of forms within this world, gross and subtle, depends on the rate and amplitude of the vibrational energy that constitutes an object or thoughts, or feeling. Instead of absorbing the *prana* in a solid form, self-realized yogis eat the vibrational energy in a finer, invisible form.

At the final stage, saints and mystics are capable of living upon "Light" alone. Jesus fasted forty days in the desert. An amazing example of this power in the West has been Therese Neumann, a Catholic German mystic, who was active and alive for many years without eating solid food.

To stop meat eating is the first step; the second is to eat pure and organic food. The third is to tune in with the Higher Divine Power that generously provides our meal. Our body is a temple, our home, the place where we live night and day and where we have the great opportunity of becoming spiritually realized. We are what we eat and we become what we eat. The body should become a clean, well-lighted place. Everything we put in our mouth will sooner or later affect the life and nature of our cells and organs. The quality of the food modifies the stability and vibrations of the total organism. If we daily eat dead bodies, corpses deprived of *pranic* energy, we damage ourselves not only physically but also mentally and spiritually as well. So, if we want to live long, very long, we must carefully select our food, preferring light, healthy, fresh, unadulterated and easy to digest vegetarian food. I also suggest transforming the kitchen to a clean, spiritual place where cooking is an art, performed with love and devotion.

Before eating, you may offer the food to God with gratitude and ask for blessings. While eating, be aware of the intrinsic value of such a powerful, divine gift. A new atmosphere of such purified lunches and dinners is very conducive for meditation, spiritual awakening and joyous exchange among peaceful, loving human beings. There is an ancient Sufi saying explaining the correlation between the mood of the meal and the digestion: "If you eat with anger, the food turns into poison."

So, if you thankfully eat pure meals, prepared with love and devotion, you can easily imagine what life could be.

Deepak Chopra, the famous vegetarian doctor and author of many best sellers, gives nine important tips for staying young:

1) Listen to your body wisdom signal for comfort and discomfort.
2) Live in the present, for this is the only moment you have. Keep your attention to what is here and now.
3) Take time to be silent, to meditate, to quiet the internal dialogue.
4) Relinquish your need for external approval.
5) When you find yourself reacting with anger or opposition to any person or circumstance, realize that you are only struggling with yourself.
6) Know that the world "out there" reflects your reality "in here."
7) Shed the burden of judgment, you will feel much lighter.
8) Don't contaminate your body with toxins, either through food, drink, or toxic emotions.
9) Replace fear-motivated behavior with love-motivated behavior. Fear is the product of memory, which dwells in the past.

Prana

The following is a quick explanation of a yoga exercise and the benefits of the absorption of *prana,* given by the yogi Sri Ganapathi Sachchidananda Swamiji:

> In our daily life, our breath control is very important. Long breath, long life. Short breath, short life. Dogs have a short breath. Therefore they have a short life. Breathing is very important. A long breath, a long *pranayama,* is beneficial for our nervous system and mental balance. When you are doing some work, a long breath is very important. Whoever practices long

breathing will not be tired at all. Many people wonder to themselves, "What is this tiredness?" Some people are always crying. Why are they crying? They don't know the reason. There is only one very important reason for all this distress: they have no long breath! That is the reason. You test long breath, you practice. Automatically, the crying and the unhappiness are controlled. That is the effect of long breath, or *pranayama. Pranayama* is very important. Yogis, the yogis in the Himalayas and the ancient yogis, Lord Jesus Christ, Saints, all have long breath. *Prana* (vital energy) is very important in yoga, *prana* is in our breathing. When some pains come in your body, you can breathe a long breath. Long inhale and long exhale. Those who use a long inhale and a long exhale live 100, 120 and 200 years. Certain yogis lived 200 or 300 years. This is from controlling our food, controlling our breathing, controlling our senses. Long breathing and high thinking. If you face trouble, sometimes sit for five minutes, practice *pranayama* and make a decision. It will give you success. It is truth. It is not a miracle. It is not magic.

Restore Health

"A suitable vegetarian diet can restore health at any age," reveals the Ayurveda. The Ayurveda is part of one of the four Vedas, the Atharva Veda, written more than 5,000 years ago. The Ayurveda contains the supreme knowledge and highest philosophy about the Science of Life. Thousands of years ago in India it was known that illness was caused by a multitude of minute, invisible creatures, today called "germs." They also knew the right use of plants and herbs to cure any disease.

The Death Rate

"In Denmark, blockaded by the Allies as a result of World War I, the death rate fell to its lowest level in 20 years by over thirty percent, when virtually the entire country was placed on a lacto-vegetarian diet."

—Keith Akers, *A Vegetarian Sourcebook*, Vegetarian Press, Box 10238, Arlington, VA 22210

Fasting

Fasting can be a very powerful healing factor. However, since no one gains any monetary profit from it, it is not advertised by any company or suggested by any group of physicians. Everybody can live one or two days without solid food. Fasting shouldn't be considered a special or strange kind of cure but the most universal and natural "remedy." To miss solid food for one day can prevent many disorders, because undigested food is one of the main causes of disease. When fasting, be sure to drink sufficient amounts of pure water. A minimum of eight glasses of water a day should be maintained at all times, especially during a fast from food. Persons with special diets, such as diabetics or those with protein-metabolizing issues, should check with their doctor before fasting. The science of nutrition teaches that periodic fasting greatly benefits the body by giving the digestive organs a rest, allowing for internal cleansing. The body then functions much more efficiently.

The body can very easily eliminate the mucus, waste and toxins accumulated day after day. Overeating is becoming a social disease and an economic disaster, ruining the health of millions. The food companies cannot appreciate any promotion of this powerful solution. There is much fear and misconception about fasting. One reason for the dizziness and weakness associated with fasting is that all the negative toxins that the body has collected from years of eating processed meat products goes into the blood circulation to be eliminated, and the symptoms created can seem like an illness. However, the body is cleansing itself as the toxins are actually exiting the body. When the

waste products are eliminated, you will feel lighter and more ener-
getic. Take the good habit to fast regularly. I suggest fasting according
to the moon. In India, since ancient times, religious people fast on
Ekadasi, which is the eleventh day of the waxing and waning moon,
approximately twice a month. Ekadasi is a day of purification regularly observed by those who follow Sanatana Dharma, or Krishna
Consciousness. Other Eastern cultures and religions also teach fasting
from both a spiritual and physical perspective, but always with the
idea of purifying the body, mind and spirit.

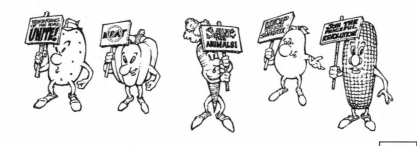

7

Vegetarianism And
World Religions

If we define religion as the best way to approach and love God, it is inconceivable to see religious people eating meat. "Any religion," said Nobel Prize winner Albert Schweitzer, "which is not based on a respect for life is not a true religion.... Until he extends his circle of compassion to all living things, man will not find peace."

Peter Singer, professor of philosophy at Monash University in Australia, explains that "The exploitation of animals is incompatible with any religion which professes compassion. There are many quotes in all the major religions about vegetarianism and it is difficult to accept the point that God created wonderful and sensitive creatures just for the slaughterhouses." The Hindus, Buddhists and Jains are all vegetarians and believe that if we are cruel to animals, we shall take an animal body in our next life to go through the same experience as the harmed animal. The majority of Christians want to believe (for how long?) that the commandment "Thou shalt not kill" is applicable only to human beings, not to animals. The Bible and Jesus didn't use the word murder, because that word only refers to human beings. The real meaning of "Thou shalt not kill" refers to any being, human or not.

You may follow some forms of religious principles, appreciate love, peace and harmony, and are non-violent to other humans—but maybe have been an unconscious meat eater for years. Now, open your heart and look at the anxiety of these poor, innocent creatures. Do you not feel the need to give them hope and add to your civilized, democratic, Declaration of Independence that all living entities are endowed, by God, the natural right to life?

Vegetarian Jews

"I've always had the feeling that Judaism's message and religious practices in general can help with all of the problems facing the world: the environment, world hunger, the arms race. Vegetarianism is consistent with Jewish ideals and can play an important role in fighting those problems."

—Richard Schwartz, author of *Judaism and
Vegetarianism*, Micah Publications

Vegetarian Jews look to inspirational leaders like the philosopher Martin Buber and the great Rabbi Abraham Isaac Kook, the first chief rabbi of pre-state Israel and a well-known scholar who firmly believed that a merciful God would not create a permanent law permitting the killing of animals for food. Rabbi Kook, who was also author of *A Vision of Peace and Vegetarianism*, wrote: "It is inconceivable that the Creator who had planned a world of harmony and a perfect way for man to live should, many thousands of years later, find that this plan was wrong."

"The practice of vegetarianism is implicit in the teachings of Judaism and is evident from the often repeated phrases in Genesis: 'to man and all creatures wherein there is a living soul.' This indicates a common life and a shared destiny and the principle is exemplified throughout biblical writings. Nowhere it is stated that abundance of flesh shall be the reward for observing the Law; rather, there are promises of fruits of the vine and pomegranates, wheat, barley and oil, and peace when each man shall sit under the shade of his own fig tree, not under the shadow of his own slaughterhouse."

—Philip L. Pick, founder of the International
Jewish Vegetarian Society

Paradise Is Vegetarian

Rashi (Rabbi Solomon von Isaac, 1030- 1105), the famous Jewish Bible commentator, taught that "God didn't permit Adam and his wife to kill a creature and to eat its flesh. Only every green herb shall they all eat together." Many prestigious Jewish biblical commentators agree with this interpretation.

The Talmud says: "Adam and many generations that followed him were strict flesh-abstainers." Moses Maimonides (1135-1204), Judaism's most influential theologian, taught that meat was prohibited because living creatures possess a degree of spiritual superiority, resembling the souls of rational beings. "It appears that the first intention of the Maker was to have men live on a strictly vegetarian diet," wrote Rabbi Simon Glazer in his *Guide to Judaism* (1971).

In the Garden of Eden and the Paradise there is no killing. All the different species live peacefully together. It appears that before the Flood the human diet was vegetarian and life spans were normally measured in terms of centuries. Adam was 930 years old. His son Seth lived up to 912. Seth's son, Enoch, lived to be 905 years old. His son, Kenan, lived to 910—all the way to the most famous, Methuselah, whose name has come to be a synonym for old age, who lived to 969. After the great devastating Flood, when for the first time meat eating became a common habit, humans decreased dramatically their life force and life spans dropped precipitously up to the present time. Abraham lived 175, far beyond today's average, but not much compared to his forebears.

"People lived the longest," noted Richard Schwartz in *Judaism and Vegetarianism*, "when they were vegetarian in the Bible."

When most of the plants were destroyed, meat eating was a concession out of necessity. Later the sacrifice of animals became a religious practice, and the corrupt and degraded priestly class found some justification to the killing, twisting the Scriptures. The joyous and pure atmosphere of the Garden of Eden became an old memory.

Vegetarianism and Early Christianity

"Killing, roasting, and devouring animals took place in the Temple at that time, in the guise of religious ceremonies. It was precisely this practice in the Temple of Jerusalem that so offended Jesus that he whipped the money changers out of the Temple, and charged them: 'How dare you make my Father's house a place of merchandise?' Not only were doves bought and sold, but animals of all kinds and sizes—killed on the spot, then roasted and eaten voraciously by the priests and their followers. The altars were covered with blood and corpses, and the air filled with the screaming of slaughtered animals. Early Christian Fathers called this custom 'diabolical'. Later, this practice was taken out of the temples and carried on in the slaughterhouse. It was made secular, removed from religious ceremonies, and out of sight of the flesh eaters. And that is precisely what we have today, worldwide."

> —Bianca Leonardo, minister of the Essene Church of Christ, in the Introduction to Upton Clary Ewing's *The Prophet of the Dead Sea Scrolls*

According to Ewing, the Nazarenes, the Ebionites, the Palestine Christians and the "Sect of the Scrolls" were one and the same people. New evidence is presented about the eating habits of those groups, and the intensely humane and all loving attitude of Jesus is described as He sets forth to fulfill the Prophet's plea for "mercy instead of sacrifice" (Hosea 6:6, Matthew 12:7).

The debate about meat eating versus vegetarianism was widespread in the early Church. The statement of St. Paul in Letters to the Corinthians is clear: "Wherefore, if meat makes my brother to offend, I will eat no flesh while the world standeth, lest I make my brother to offend.

The earliest Christians were vegetarians. Clemens Prudentius, the first Christian hymn writer, exhorts his fellow Christians in one of his hymns not to pollute their hands and hearts by the slaughter of innocent cows. Vasu Murty's research, published as *A Guide to Interreligious Understanding*, gives some evidence that early Christians were vegetarians:

> Seneca (5 B.C.- A.D. 65), a leading stoic philosopher and a tutor of Nero, was an ardent vegetarian. He

started a vegetarian movement during one of Rome's
most decadent periods. Christians were vegetarians,
so the Emperor became suspicious that Seneca might
also be a Christian, so he went back to eating animal
flesh. Pliny, who was Governor of Bithynia, where
Peter had preached, wrote a letter to Trajan, the Roman
Emperor, describing the early Christian practices:
"They met on a day before it was light (before sunrise)
and addressed a form of prayer to Christ, binding
themselves by a solemn oath never to commit any sin
or evil and never to falsify their word, nor deny a trust,
after which it was their custom to meet together again
to take food, but ordinary and innocent."

The original teachings of Jesus correspond to the visions of peace and
vegetarianism given in Genesis by God Himself. If you are an honest
and sincere Christian, go back to your roots and give up the unnatural
eating of meat.

"And to every beast of the earth, and to every fowl of the air, and
to every thing that creepeth upon the earth, wherein there is life, I have
given every green herb for meat: and it was so. And God saw everything that He had made and behold, it was good."
—Genesis 1: 30-31

"Plant life, instead of animal food, is the keystone of regeneration.
Jesus used bread instead of flesh and wine in place of blood at the
Lord's Supper."
—Richard Wagner (1813-1883),
German Composer

No Blood

"But flesh with the life thereof, which is the blood thereof, shall ye
not eat."
—Genesis 9:4

The Forbidden Food

"Even into modern times, the scientists' love for the taste of meat prevents them from analyzing what a foreign diet does to the brain of a herbivore. For any analysis which would determine that it is destructive to the normal physiologic function of the brain would force them to give up eating one of their favorite foods. They would be unable to escape the conclusion that what they enjoy most harms them most. So we are no better off than the recorder of the ancient fable preserved for us in Genesis. We would much rather perpetuate the error and keep the forbidden food a symbolic 'apple' than for it to be the ever present center of almost every meal: MEAT."

—Charles P. Vaclavik,
The Vegetarianism of Jesus Christ

Eat From The Table of God

"Let us therefore follow after the things which make peace, and things wherewith one may edify another. Take care not to destroy God's work for the sake of something to eat. It is good neither to eat flesh, nor to drink wine, nor any thing whereby thy brother stumbleth or is offended or is made weak."

—Romans 14:19-21

"So eat always from the table of God: the fruits of the trees, the grain and grasses of the field, the milk of beasts, and the honey of bees. For everything beyond these is of Satan, and leads by the way of sins and of diseases unto death. But the foods which you eat from the abundant table of God give strength and youth to your body, and you will never see disease. For the table of God fed Methuselah of old, and I tell you truly, if you live even as he lived, then will the God of the living give you also long life upon the earth as was his. For I tell you truly, the God of the living is richer than all the rich of the earth, and His abundant table is richer than the richest table of feasting of all the rich upon the Earth. Eat, therefore, all your life at the table of our Earthly Mother."

—from *The Essene Gospel of Peace*, third-century
Aramaic manuscript, edited and translated by

Edmond Bordeaux Szekely, co-founder with
Nobel Prize winner for Literature Romain
Rolland of the International Biogenic Society,
Apartado 372, Cartago, Costa Rica, Central
America

Don't Follow

If everybody around you is eating meat, what to do? Remember
the Bible!
"Do not follow the majority when they do evil."
—Exodus 23:2

Back to Eden

"The whole fabric of Christian 'agape' is woven from the threads
of sacrificial acts. To abstain, on principle, from eating animals, therefore, although it is not the end-all, can be the begin-all of our consci-
entious effort to journey back to Eden, can be one way (among others)
to re-establish or create that relationship to the earth which, if Genesis
1 is to be trusted, was part of God's original hopes for and plans in
creation. It is the integrity of this creation we seek to understand and
aspire to honor. In the choice of our food, I believe, we see, not in a
glass darkly, but face to face, a small but not unimportant part of both
the challenge and the promise of Christianity and animal rights."
    —from a speech by Tom Regan, author of *The
    Case for Animal Rights* before the Conference
    on Creation Theology and Environmental
    Ethics at the World Council of Churches,
    Annecy, France (September 1988)

Return to the Garden

"God Almighty first planned a Garden, and indeed it is the purest
of human pleasure."
    —Francis Bacon, *Essays,* 1625

Steven Rosen, author of *Diet for Transcendence*, points out that the older a religion is, the closer it is to vegetarian principles: "Kindness to all creatures is a fundamental religious tenet that sort of gets lost over the years. From the total vegetarian Hinduism, more than 5000 years old, to the most recent 1300-year-old Islam, the vegetarian practice gets lost even if there are bases in the Scriptures."

"The Bible, while it was inspired by God, was written by the people," says Mary Aktay, a vegetarian and director of communications for the Roman Catholic Diocese of Paterson, N.J. "Just as history is written in the words of the conquerors, the Bible was written by the people in power at the time. If you've got a monk someplace who loves his roast beef and mutton, he is not going to be too enamored of Jesus the vegetarian."

Whoever has a sincere desire to follow God's Plan and restore His Kingdom on this planet Earth should become vegetarian. Then guide others to pursue this noble vision. It is very difficult, almost impossible, for an intelligent and compassionate person to even conceive the idea that God is so cruel that He blesses or accepts the slaughtering of his dear creatures.

The orthodox, fourth-century Christian Hieronimus connected vegetarianism with both the original diet given by God and with the teachings of Jesus: "The eating of animal meat was unknown up to the Flood, but since the Flood they have pushed the strings and stinking juices of animal meat into our mouths, just as they threw quails in front of the grumbling sensual people in the desert. Jesus Christ, who appeared when the time has been fulfilled, has again joined the end with the beginning, so that it is no longer allowed for us to eat animal meat."

Jesus Was Vegetarian

"For I tell you truly, he who kills, kills himself, and whosoever eats the flesh of slain beasts eats the body of death."
—Jesus Christ, *The Essene Gospel of Peace*

In his excellent book, *Famous Vegetarians*, Rynn Berry includes Lord Jesus Christ in the list of great vegetarians:

Although the evidence for Jesus' vegetarianism is largely circumstantial, however, it is nonetheless compelling. Even Dr. Hugh Schonfield, writing in *The Passover Plot*—probably the most rigorous and demythologized life of Jesus ever written—asserts that Jesus belonged to a strict vegetarian branch of the Essenes in northern Judea—the Nazarenes. Schonfield writes: "The name borne by the earliest followers of Jesus was not Christians, they were called 'Nazarenes', and Jesus himself was known as the Nazarene.

Another interesting reading is *The Vegetarianism of Jesus Christ* by Charles P. Vaclavik. The author shows historical evidence from the writings of the early Catholic Fathers, the Jewish historian Josephus, and the Jewish philosopher Philo that Jesus and his disciples were not only vegetarians, but they also taught the practice to their followers. The book is published by Kaweah Publishing Company, P.O. Box 118, Platteville, WI 53818.

And from *The Higher Taste*, Bhaktivedanta Book Trust:

Major stumbling blocks for many Christians are the belief that Christ ate meat and the many references to meat in the New Testament. But close study of the original Greek manuscripts shows that the vast majority of the words translated as "meat" are *trophe, brome* and other words that simply mean "food" or "eating" in the broadest sense. For example, in the Gospel of St. Luke (8:55), we read that Jesus raised a woman from the dead and "commanded to give her meat." The original Greek word translated as "meat" is *phago*, which means only "to eat." So, what Christ actually said was, "let her eat." The Greek word for meat is *kreas* (flesh), and it is never used in connection with Christ. Nowhere in the New Testament is there any direct reference to Jesus eating meat. This is in line with Isaiah's famous prophecy about Jesus's appearance:

> "Behold, a virgin shall conceive , and bear a son, and
> shall call his name Immanuel. Butter and honey shall
> he eat, that he may know to refuse the evil and choose
> the good."

The Bible is the work of many hands and food is not the only subject
for which there are contradictory messages in different sections. The
discovery of earlier versions of the ancient text has led some scholars
to believe that some wordings may have been errors in translation.
Steven Rosen counts 19 references to "meat" in the English translation of the Gospels. Studying original Greek texts, he says, reveals that
a better translation would be "food", as in Matthew 25:35: "For I was
hungered, and ye gave me meat; I was thirsty, and ye gave me drink."

"The Greek words are usually *broma* meaning "food"; *brosis,*
"food or the act of eating"; *trophe,* "nourishment", and so on . The
King James Bible, an English translation in common use, was written
in 1611. At that time, the expression "meat and drink" was a common
way to refer to a meal, whether it included flesh or not."

—Max Friedman, "Food of the Gods," published
in *Vegetarian Times*

John the Baptist Was Vegetarian

We read in the Gospel of Matthew 3:4, "And the same John had
his raiment of camel's hair, and a leathern girdle about his loins: and
his food was locusts and wild honey." John was a great saint and vegetarian, the word "locusts" doesn't refer to the insects but to the locust
beans, or carob, also known as "St. John's bread".

READ THE BIBLE AND REMEMBER
THE SIXTH COMMANDMENT
"Thou shalt not kill."

The New Catholic Catechism

Following centuries of ruthless, dogmatic and cruel humanocentrism, the Catholic Church continues the old policy of animal slaughtering. We read in the *Catechism of the Catholic Church* (from the official English translation, published by Geoffrey Chapman, London, June 1994) that animals are good for food: "God entrusted animals to the stewardship of those whom he created in his own image. Hence it is legitimate to use animals for food and clothing or they may be domesticated to help man in his work and leisure."

What then must be done? Leave the Catholic Church with her anti-progressive, unenlightened views on animals, or express openly your opposition to the higher authorities? Being free to express your views openly and honestly is a human right...use that right.

The author of *Christianity and the Rights of Animals*, Rev. Professor Andrew Linzey, holds the world's first academic post in theology and animal welfare at Mansfield College, University of Oxford. He suggests that all who care for animals should communicate their concern and complaints to the Church. "Catholics should make their views in writing to their priest, bishop, archbishop and to the Pope himself. It is also vital that letters are published in the religious press engendering Church debate about animals. Others need also to write to the Catholic hierarchy to make known their disappointment and sadness at the failure of the Church to take a moral stand."

Steven Rosen, author of *Diet for Transcendence*, explains the old battle inside the Church about animals:

> ...over the centuries, there has arisen two distinct schools of Christian thought. The Aristotelian-Thomistic school and the Augustinian-Franciscan school. The Aristotelian-Thomistic school has, as its fundamental basis, the premise that animals are here for our pleasure—they have no purpose of their own. We can eat them, torture them in laboratories—anything...

Unfortunately, modern Christianity   embraces this
form of their religion. The Augustinian-Franciscan
school, however, teaches that we are all brothers and
sisters under God's Fatherhood. Based largely on the
world view of St. Francis and being platonic in nature,
this school fits very neatly with the vegetarian
perspective.

The fact that humans were made in God's image and given
"dominion" over all creation, including animals, does not justify the
killing of animals; God Himself gave, very clearly, in Genesis, plants
as food. The big misunderstanding is about the word "dominion".

Dr. Michael Fox, vice-president of the Humane Society, has
explained that the word "dominion" is derived from the original
Hebrew word *rahe,* which refers to compassionate relation and care,
instead of heavy power and brutal control. He gives the example of the
family—if parents have dominion over their children, that doesn't
allow them to abuse, exploit, torture or kill them. The Talmud
(Shabbat 119; Sanhedrin 7) allows dominion over animals only for
labor.

The Code of Law

The ancient Indian philosophy emphasized the spiritual conception of the unity of all life. As Bhaktivedanta Swami Prabhupada
writes:

In the *Manu-samhita* the concept of a life for a life is
sanctioned, and it is actually observed throughout the
world. Similarly, there are other laws which state that
one cannot even kill an ant without being responsible.
Since we cannot create, we have no right to kill any
living entity, and therefore man-made laws that distin-
guish between killing a man and killing an animal are
imperfect....

According to the laws of God, killing an animal is as
punishable as killing a man. Those who draw distinc-

tions between the two are concocting their own laws. Even in the Ten Commandments, it is prescribed, "Thou shalt not kill." This is a perfect law, but by discriminating and speculating men distort it. "I shall not kill man, but I shall kill animals." In this way people cheat themselves and inflict suffering on themselves and others. Everyone is God's creature, although in different bodies or dresses. God is considered the one Supreme Father. A father may have many children, and some may be intelligent and others not very intelligent, but if an intelligent son tells his father, "My brother is not very intelligent; let me kill him," will the father agree?...

Similarly, if God is the Supreme Father, why should He sanction the killing of animals who are also His sons?

The Oldest Teachings

The Mahabharata, the epic poem of India that contains 100,000 verses and is said to be the longest and oldest poem in the world, tells us:

Who can be more cruel and selfish than he who augments his flesh by eating the flesh of innocent animals?

He who desires to increase the flesh of his own body by eating the flesh of other creatures lives in misery in whatever species he may take his birth.

Those who desire to possess good memory, beauty, long life with perfect health, and physical, moral and spiritual strength should abstain from animal food.

The Law of Karma

"He who does not seek to cause the suffering of bonds and death to living creatures, but desires the good of all beings, obtains endless bliss. He who does not injure any creature attains without any effort what he thinks of, what he undertakes, and what he fixes his mind on. Meat can never be obtained without injury to living creatures, and injury to sentient beings is detrimental to the attainment of heavenly bliss; let him therefore shun the use of meat. Having well considered the disgusting origin of flesh and the cruelty of fettering and slaying of corporeal beings, let him entirely abstain from eating flesh. He who does not eat meat becomes dear to men, and will not be tormented by diseases. He who permits the slaughter of an animal, he who cuts it up, he who kills it, he who buys or sells meat, he who cooks it, he who serves it up, and he who eats it—all must be considered as the slayers of the animal. There is no greater sinner than that man who seeks to increase his own flesh by the flesh of other beings."
—The Law of Manu 5:46-52

Useless killing of innocent animals will only generate bad karma, bad reactions. Many world religions respect life and believe that those who kill will be killed. The law of karma is absolutely scientific and should be explained in detail even to small children. Karma is a natural principle, a scientific and cosmic law, which means cause and effect. When we understand that any action generates a reaction, we finally see how this cruel slaughtering can badly damage our future. When you, or somebody on your behalf, kills another entity, we contaminate our life and the bad effects will strike back and hit us, sooner or later, in this life or the next. There is no injustice in the universe; whoever violates this sacred spiritual principle of life will get a proportionate reaction.

Please get rid of this bad, "non-human" habit and improve the quality of your existence. No one can escape the negative consequences of the law of karma except those who fully understand how it works. Vegetarianism can help you reach higher spiritual dimensions and re-develop a natural appreciation and love for God. The ancient Vedas explain that human beings are meant for spiritual life, and for that purpose they shouldn't eat anything that is not first offered to the

Lord. How can you offer to God pieces of a dead body? That in itself creates bad karma.

The Scientific Effects of Karma

Those who kill animals and give them unnecessary pain—as people do in slaughterhouses—will be killed in a similar way in the next life and in many lives to come. In the Judeo-Christian scriptures, it is stated clearly: Thou shalt not kill!

"Nonetheless, giving all kinds of excuses, even the heads of religion indulge in killing animals and at the same time try to pass as saintly persons. This mockery and hypocrisy in human society brings about unlimited calamities such as great wars, where masses of people go out onto the battlefields and kill each other."
—Bhaktivedanta Swami Prabhupada

Your Eating Habits Can Affect Your Next Incarnation

"All men tremble at punishment, all men fear death: remember that you are like unto them, and do not kill, nor cause slaughter. All men tremble at punishment, all men love life; remember that thou art like unto them, and do not kill, nor cause slaughter. He who, seeking his own happiness, punishes or kills beings who also long for happiness, will not find happiness after death."
—Dhammapada 10:129

The ancient Veda speaks very clear about the scientific law of karma and reincarnation: "The living entity, who has received his present body because of his past fruitive activity, by performing actions in this present life determines his next body." More than 5000 years ago *Srimad Bhagavatam* warned people about their habits, especially about food. It is just a popular myth that the soul, once attaining a human form, always comes back in a human body in the next life and never reincarnates in lower species. The book, *Coming Back: The*

Science of Reincarnation, published by the Bhaktivedanta Book Trust, points out that

> We may reincarnate as human, but we could come back as dogs, pigs, chickens, hogs or lower species. The soul, however, despite entering higher or lower bodies, remains unchanged. In any case, the type of body one gets in his next life will be determined by the type of consciousness he develops in this life and by the immutable law of karma. *Bhagavad-gita*, the most authoritative sourcebook on reincarnation, spoken by God Himself, clearly states that when one dies in the mode of ignorance, he takes birth in the animal kingdom. There is no scientific or scriptural evidence anywhere for this fanciful "once a human always a human" notion, which runs contrary to the true principles of reincarnation, principles that have been understood and followed by millions of people since time immemorial.

Meditate on the fact that the path of reincarnation does not always lead uphill; now you are in a human body but are always the eternal spirit soul residing inside. In your next life you may enter another body, but human birth is not guaranteed. Multiple karmic reactions secondary to your disrespectful activity can cause you serious problems. Respect for life and animals will make your life more spiritually prosperous and easier. Be vegetarian. Offer your food to God and feed the people less fortunate than yourself and your life will become more complete. This activity is karma-free and is sure to keep your spiritual growth on an upward path.

Meditate On The Bad Karma

There are 1.8 billion domesticated mammals killed for human consumption every year, along with 22.5 billion birds, chicken and other poultry, and trillions of fishes. In the U.S. alone more than 120 million farm animals a week are killed for food. Add hundreds of millions of innocent animals tortured in medical research laboratories (every three seconds an animal dies in an American laboratory) or slaughtered for their fur, hide, skin or hunted for sport. Meditate on these numbers and guess: Who is going to pay the heavy karmic bill? Who will get the reactions? Do something to stop this crime now. Be a good human being!

Buddha Was Vegetarian

"He who causes suffering shall suffer. There is no escape."
—Buddha

"The eating of meat extinguishes the seed of great compassion."
—Mahaparinirvana Sutra

"To avoid causing terror to living beings, let the disciple refrain from eating meat . . . the food of the wise is that which is consumed by the sadhus (holy men); it does not consist of meat....There may be some foolish people in the future who will say that I permitted meat-eating and that I partook of meat myself, but...meat-eating I have not permitted to anyone, I do not permit, I will not permit meat-eating in any form, in any manner or in any place; it is unconditionally prohibited for all."
—Buddha, from the Dhammapada

From "*The Key to Immediate Enlightenment*" by Supreme Master Ching Hai:

Question: A long time ago I heard another Master say, "Buddha ate a pig's foot and then got diarrhea and died." It is true?

Answer: Absolutely not. It was because of eating a kind of mushroom that Buddha died.

If we translate directly from the language of the Brahmans, this kind of mushroom is called the "pig's foot", but it is not a real pig's foot. It's just like when we call a kind of fruit *longan* (in Chinese this literally means the "dragon's eye"). There are many things that by name are not vegetables but actually are vegetarian food, such things as the "dragon's eye". This mushroom in Brahmanic language is called "pig's foot" or "pig's joy".

Both have a connection with pigs. This kind of mushroom was not easy to find in ancient India and was a rare delicacy, so people offered it to Buddha in worship. This mushroom cannot be found above the ground. It grows under the ground. If people want to find it they must search with the help of an old pig which likes very much to eat this kind of mushroom. Pigs detect by their smell, and when they discover one, they use their feet to dig in the mud to find and eat it. That was why this kind of mushroom is called the "pig's joy" or "pig's foot". Actually these two names refer to the same mushroom. Because it was translated carelessly and because people did not truly understand the derivation, following generations have misunderstood and mistake Buddha for a "flesh devouring man". This is really a regrettable thing.

Lord Buddha was openly against animal sacrifice and meat eating, his important preaching of *ahimsa* (nonviolence) became part of the Indian tradition as a fundamental step on the path of spiritual realization and self-awareness. He said to his followers: "Do not butcher the ox that plows the fields." and "Do not indulge a voracity that involves the slaughter of animals."

"I do not see any reason why animals should be slaughtered to serve as human diet when there are so many substitutes. After all, man can live without meat..."
—The Dalai Lama

Was Mohammed Vegetarian?

"If you read the life of Mohammed carefully," says Steven Rosen, author of *Diet for Transcendence*, "he really seems to be someone who does have compassion for animals."

The Prophet of Islam said, "Verily God is more compassionate on his creatures than a woman on her own child." and "Whoever is kind to the creatures of God is kind to himself."

"There is not an animal on earth, nor a flying creature flying on two wings, but they are peoples like unto you."
—Koran, Surah 6, verse 38

Sikhs

Guru Nanak Dev, the founder of the Sikhism, consumed only vegetarian food, and the prasad distributed in Gurudwara Temples is always vegetarian.

Jains

The Jains are total vegetarians and claim that their principles of *ahimsa* (nonviolence) have inspired all other Buddhist and Hindu groups. Often they cover their mouth, trying to avoid breathing in insects. "Like the Pythagoreans," writes Rynn Berry in *Famous Vegetarians*, "the Jains were great mathematicians and astronomers. They are credited with having invented the concept of infinity."

Speciesism: The Last Barrier!

"Speciesism"—a new term—entered our language only a few years ago. The dictionary says it is 1) a prejudice or attitude of bias toward the interests of members of one's own species and against those of members of another species, 2) a word used to describe the widespread discrimination that is practiced by "Homo Sapiens" against the other species. Philospher Peter Singer defines speciesism as allowing the interest of one's own species "to override the greater interest of other species."

Speciesism is an evil like all other historical prejudices, such as racism, sexism, sectarianism, nationalism or classism. After many centuries of constant battles for freedom, intelligent people have come to understand that skin color, gender, class, religion and other classifications are irrelevant when it comes to granting equal rights and protection to humans. Now speciesism is the last barrier of our culture, the obstacle to remove to start a real civilization. There is no moral justification to our society's exploitation, harming and killing of animals. The differences between humans and nonhumans can't be used as an excuse.

"Speciesism is so ingrained in our culture," explains the *Antivivisection* magazine, "that it is convenient to believe that species difference is a relevant criteria for granting protection. In fact, our acceptance of speciesism is so widespread that we allow animals to be mutilated and killed for many reasons—to test cosmetics, please our taste buds, entertain us and satisfy our curiosity in research labs. But it does not have to be so. We can choose to live by an ethic which exploits neither people nor animals."

So you are invited to become an active member of the movement ending speciesism. Mankind needs to make another final step towards a more compassionate world, in which people love animals instead of exploiting or abusing them. Remind your fellow humans that humans are not the only species on earth, even if they act as if they are.

A New Species Consciousness

"By eliminating beef from the human diet, our species takes a significant step forward to a new species consciousness, reaching out in a spirit of shared partnership with the bovine, and by extension, other sentient creatures with whom we share the earth."
—Jeremy Rifkin, *Beyond Beef*

What Do You Need To Know If You Are Vegetarian And Want To Have Vegetarian Pets?

We recommend the book by James A. Peden, *Vegetarian Cats & Dogs*. Peden has, since 1986, published books documenting research and experience with vegetarian pets. The Executive Director of the International Veterinary Acupuncture Society, David H. Jaggar (MRCVS,DC), writes: "*Vegetarian Cats & Dogs* is a solid work of ethical integrity and is meritorious as an example of applying scientific information to progressive ends. The scientific rationale is as sound as the moral arguments are incisive and persuasive. The author is sincere in his commitment to a scientifically sound means to feed dogs and cats with superior nourishment (meeting all the known nutritional requirements for different stages of life), while at the same time reducing large scale animal suffering in agribusiness."

Feed your companion animals as family members, and just see how much they appreciate and reward your efforts in providing them with fresh food. Prepare meals ahead of time in your own kitchen using freshly obtained ingredients, such as garbanzo beans, high protein flour, corn flour and food yeast.

For more information and to place an order of vegetarian food for cats and dogs, contact: Harbingers of a New Age, 717 E. Missoula Avenue, Troy MT 59935-9609. Fax 406/295-7603, Support 406/295-4944, Toll Free for orders: 800/884-6262

"If, for any reason, you are seeking to feed your companion animal a healthier diet, free from the products of the slaughterhouse, then *Vegetarian Cats & Dogs* should be considered required reading."
—Michael Klaper, MD, author and lecturer

Stay Vegetarian, Check The Dictionary

You can eat animals without knowing. Animal-based ingredients can be lurking in the most obscure way, in a variety of food and other products. With strange technical names like pepsin, casein, urea and tallowate, you'd need a dictionary to investigate all of the terms. To help you find some of the answers you are looking for, take a look at

A Consumer's Dictionary of Food Additives by Ruth Winter, MS, 1994. This book provides definitions and explanations for thousands of additives. You can find it in major bookstores or libraries.

Thought-Provoking Facts About Vegetarianism

Fourteen million Americans are now vegetarian and over 30 million are exploring a diet with little use of meat.

Percentage of illnesses that could be delayed or eliminated just by dietary changes: 50%

Amount the U.S. Government spends annually on price supports for beef and veal: $10 billion

Amount of cropland producing livestock feed: 64%

Amount of U.S. cropland producing fruits and vegetables: 2%

Water needed to produce 1 pound of meat: 2500 gallons

Water needed to produce 1 pound of wheat: 25 gallons

Amount of U.S. topsoil lost from cropland, pasture, rangeland and forest land directly associated with livestock raising: 85%

Historic cause of demise of many great civilizations: topsoil depletion.

Amount of corn grown in U.S. consumed by human beings: 20%

Amount of corn grown in U.S. consumed by livestock: 80%

Nearly 1.5 million Americans are crippled and killed each year by diseases associated with excessive consumption of meat and animal fat. The elements held principally accountable include saturated fat, cholesterol, hormones, pesticides and nitrites.

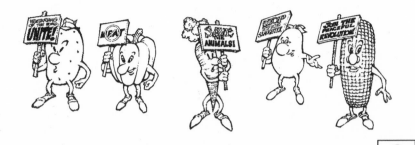

8

Open Letter
to McDonalds

I am vegetarian and right now I am not one of your clients. I visited your places a couple of times and saw that the cleanliness and the service are first class, very dynamic and efficient.

The one big problem I found is that you slaughter animals for food. If you haven't read Jeremy Rifkin's *Beyond Beef*, you should be informed that "Today, millions of Americans, Europeans and Japanese are consuming countless hamburgers, steaks and roast, oblivious to the impact their dietary habits are having on the biosphere and the very survivability of life on earth. Every pound of grain-fed flesh is secured at the expense of a burned forest, an eroded rangeland, a barren field, a dried-up river or stream, and the release of millions of tons of carbon dioxide, nitrous oxide and methane into the skies."

Diligently you keep track of the billions of hamburgers you have served all over the world. I guess they were all paid for and you made a good profit. Now I have a question for you: Who will pay the karmic bill? You? Or will you share this with your clients? The karmic bill is the unavoidable reaction to the senseless killing of innocent animals. Meditate just for one minute about LIFE. Do you want to exist and have a life? So, why should cattle not have the same right as you? Have you been made aware of the karmic consequences? Are you ready—like is done for cigarettes—to warn your clients about the negative side effects of hamburgers?

We are compassionate vegetarians; we have no enemies. We love God, we love life, we love people and we love animals, too.

Probably you have been so busy opening new spots that you never had the time to stop and consider seriously the negative impact of your huge business. We don't wish you failure. We are fully aware that thousands of employees and their families rely on you for their maintenance. If you find the time, please read *Diet for A New America*, written by John Robbins, heir to the famous family who owns the world's largest ice cream company—Baskin-Robbins. Born right in the heart of the Great American Food Machine, he had a real change of heart and, taking a distance from his family's empire, started to envision "A society at peace with its conscience because it respects and lives in harmony with all life forms. A dream of a people living in accord with the laws of Creation, cherishing and caring for the natural environment, conserving nature instead of destroying it. A dream of a society that is truly healthy, practicing a wise and compassionate stewardship of a balanced ecosystem." He wrote in his book about your business, so similar to the one of his successful family: "At the present time, when most of us sit down to eat, we aren't very aware of how food choices affect the world. We don't realize that in every Big Mac there is a piece of the tropical species become extinct. We don't realize that in the sizzle of our steaks there is the suffering of animals, the mining of our topsoil, the slashing of our forest, the harming of our economy, and the eroding of our health. We don't hear in the sizzle the cry of the hungry millions who might otherwise be fed. We don't see the toxic poisons accumulating in the food chains, poisoning our children and our earth for generations to come."

Maybe, following his footsteps, one day we will have the *McDonald's Vegetarian Cookbook* with many tasty recipes for veggie burgers.

What we suggest now is a positive shift in your eating habits. Move from the cruel and bloody meat diet to the more peaceful and civilized vegetarian diet. Knowing that you are receptive to positive messages, we wish for you a very good future.

Thomas Berry in *Befriending The Earth* puts me, you and everyone else together: "The human community and the natural world will go into the future as a single sacred community or we will both perish in the desert."

The Russian dictator Joseph Stalin used to say, "A single death is a tragedy, a million deaths is a statistic." You are, now, proud to count how many hamburgers you have sold.

For many sensitive people this is just nonstop tragedy—a sad, cruel accounting of unbearable pain and suffering. Please change your style and sell billions and billions of veggie burgers. Your consciousness will remain pure and crystal clear. Your clients and your employees will appreciate your positive transformation.

If you study history, you can see that none—not even the so-called greatest heroes and powerful leaders—could escape the reactions of their mistakes. And we can guarantee you that to serve meat is a major mistake. Remember the meat business is one of the biggest causes of such environmental problems as deforestation, desertification, and air and water pollution. The grain-fed meat industry also diverts grain from human consumption, thus contributing substantially to world hunger.

Thank you for your attention. We write you this letter knowing that you will read it and take it seriously. More than five thousand years ago, Sri Krishna spoke in the *Bhagavad-gita* about human psychology: "Whatever actions a great man performs, common men follow. And whatever standards he sets by exemplary acts, all the world pursues." You have a Great Power and a Great Name; if you are willing to make the shift, the whole world will remember McDonalds as a great well-wisher. We are ready to offer freely all possible cooperation for the wonderful transformation of your food business.

—GIORGIO CERQUETTI
President of Vegetarians International

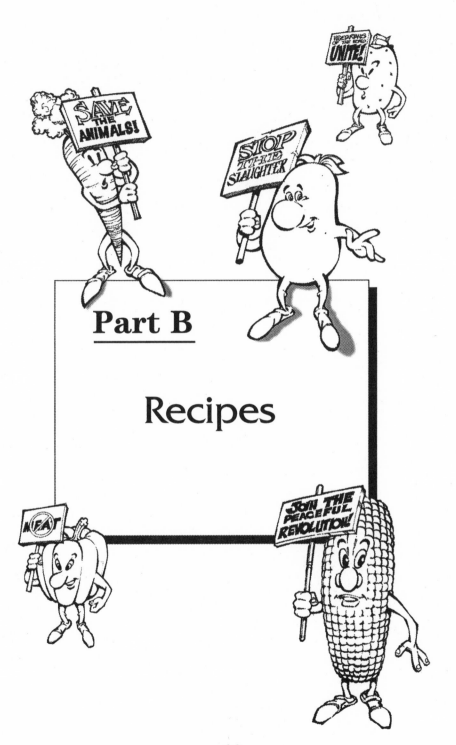

Part B

Recipes

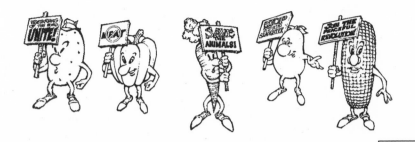

9

Recipes of
Famous People

Every day, all over the world, thousands of intelligent and sensitive people are realizing the need to improve the quality of their life, removing blood and violence from their kitchens.

Would you like to be one of them?

Giulia Amici lives in Italy. In the early 1970s, she wrote one of the first successful Italian vegetarian cookbooks, *Alimentazione Alternativa*. Currently, she promotes yoga, meditation and vegetarianism through different media.

MINESTRONE SOUP

2 tbs. olive oil
1 cup tomato (skinned and
    chopped)
1/3 cup garbanzo beans
    (soaked overnight)

1/4 cup basil leaves
1 parsley sprig (chopped)
9 cups water
1 carrot (peeled and diced)

1 celery stalk (diced)	freshly ground pepper
1 cup diced potatoes	1/2 cup barley
1 large zucchini (diced)	1/2 cup parmesan cheese
1 cup shredded cabbage	1/2 tsp. asafetida
salt	

Heat oil in large saucepan, add hing and cabbage. Sauté for 1 minute. Add tomatoes, garbanzo beans, basil, parsley, and water. Bring to a boil, cover, and simmer for 1 hour.

Add carrots and celery, and cook for 20 more minutes. Add remaining ingredients, except for cheese. Cook 45 more minutes. Add salt to taste. Let the soup stand for 15 minutes. Stir in parmesan cheese and serve hot. Serves 6.

Bawa Muhaiyaddeen
The Bawa Muhaiyaddeen Fellowship
5820 Overbrook Avenue
Philadelphia, PA 19131

This recipe has been excerpted from *Food for the Gods: Vegetarianism and the World's Religions* by Rynn Berry, Pythagorean Publishers, PO Box 8174 JAF Stn, New York, NY 10116.

Many Sufis are vegetarian and practice a peaceful spirituality. This recipe reflects their open-minded hospitality and desire to gather and serve people.

FOOD FOR THE SUFIS

Cooking time: 2 1/2 hours	40 large potatoes: quarter
Quantity: 15 gallons	lengthwise and slice thin
Ingredients for Curry	20 large carrots: quarter
16 cups great northern beans	lengthwise and slice thin
3 lb. frozen lima beans	30 small tomatoes: slice thin
3 lb. frozen peas	2 lb. string beans: cut in half
10 large onions: chop small	inch pieces

2 large cabbages: chop small
25 bell peppers: chop
oil

Method for Curry

Boil great northern beans separately till soft, about one and half hours. Drain and set aside. In 2 separate pots: boil lima beans and peas till soft. Drain and set aside. In 1 to 2 large frying pans, while beans are cooking: fill the pan with 1/4 inch oil. Heat. Add the onions and sauté till golden brown. Drain and set aside. Reuse the oil drained from the onions, and after each following batch of vegetables, add fresh oil as needed to fill the pan to 1/4 inch. Sauté each of the following vegetables till just done: potatoes, carrots, tomatoes, string beans, cabbage, cauliflower and bell peppers. Add 2 tsp. salt to each batch. Add 1 1/2 cups hot water to the potatoes only. Stir as needed, cooking on medium-high heat with lid on. Drain each batch of vegetables, except for the last, after cooking; then mix them together in even amounts in 3 large basins.

Sauce

1/2 large onion: chop	**1 heaping tbs. cumin**
10 chili peppers: chop small	**3 heaping tbs. garlic**
3 18 oz cans tomato paste	**1 1/2 tbs. ginger**
juice of 6 lemons	**9 heaping tbs. salt**
oil	**1 rounded tbs. turmeric**
	Seed spices:
Powdered spices:	**1 1/2 tsp. cumin**
1 rounded tbs. cardamom	**1 tsp. fennel**
2 rounded tbs. cayenne	**1 1/2 tsp. fenugreek**
1 1/2 tbs. cinnamon	**1 1/2 tsp. black mustard**
1 1/2 tbs. cloves	**9" stick cinnamon (broken up)**
2 heaping tbs. coriander	**1 handful curry leaves**

Method for Sauce

In a wok: Cover bottom well with oil. Heat. Add the seed spices, cinnamon sticks and curry leaves. When seeds pop, add the onions and chilies. Sauté till onions turn clear. Heat on medium, sprinkle in the powdered spices and mix well. Let simmer. Mix the tomato paste with

4 cups hot water. After spices have simmered a few minutes, add the tomato paste with 2 cups hot rinse water. Cover and continue to simmer, stirring occasionally. Five minutes later, add the lemon juice. Add hot water, if needed, to make a medium-thick sauce consistency. Cook for 10 more minutes; then pour the sauce evenly over the three basins. Mix each basin well. Salt to taste.

Annie Besant

"In the late nineteenth century Annie Besant was one of the most admired and accomplished women in the world. Striking looking physically, perspicacious mentally; versatile and many-sided professionally—in her person she gave promise of what liberated women might achieve in the twentieth century. As a publisher and editor of a widely-read Freethought journal, *Our Corner*, she was the first to recognize Shaw's genius and publish his novels in serial form. As the country's first laywoman lawyer, she trounced some of England's most respected barristers in court. As a pioneering trade unionist, she led England's first successful strike on behalf of female workers (the match girls). In 1889, after joining the Theosophical Society at the age of forty-two, she became Madame Blavatsky's heir apparent and, on the latter's death in 1891, succeeded her as the international president of the Theosophical Society, with headquarters in Adyar, India. Long before Gandhi was even so much as a mote on the political horizon, Annie had called for the Indians to throw off the British colonial yoke, and had drafted a constitution for an independent Indian government that served as a model for the one that was eventually drawn up by Nehru. Annie was elected President of the Indian National Congress, the highest elective office ever held by a Britisher in India."

—from *Famous Vegetarians* by Rynn Berry

WATERCRESS SALAD SANDWICH

1 bunch watercress, tough stems removed	4 tbs. olive oil
1/2 cup bean sprouts	1 tbs. red wine vinegar
1/2 cup halved walnuts	1 clove minced garlic
1/2 cup green onions, chopped	1/2 tsp. salt
	1/2 tsp. Dijon mustard

Toasted whole-grain bread slices, or oven-warmed whole-wheat burger buns.

Rinse the watercress and bean sprouts, pick over, and pat dry with a towel. Remove the tough stems from the watercress, and discard. Halve the walnuts and chop the onions, then set aside. In a large salad bowl, combine the last seven ingredients (excluding bread), and make a dressing. To the dressing add the watercress, halved walnuts, bean sprouts, and chopped green onions. Mix thoroughly, and serve between slices of toasted whole grain bread, or on oven-warmed whole-wheat burger buns. Serves 2.

Bhaktivedanta Swami Prabhupada, Founder-Acarya of the International Society for Krishna Consciousness.

"Ex Oriente Lux is a Latin phrase that means light (or wisdom) that comes from the East. The same might be said for the phenomenon of vegetarianism itself. The cradle of vegetarianism is India. Every philosophy or religion associated with vegetarianism has had its origin in India. Each wave of vegetarianism that has broken upon Western shores has either directly or indirectly come from India. It could be argued that the same wave that brought vegetarianism to the U.S. in the 1960s had bobbing on its surface the freighter that carried the most improbable world teacher that the West had ever known. After chugging into New York Harbor on September 19, 1965, the Indian freighter Jaladuta disgorged a most unusual passenger. Clad in a saffron-colored dhoti and chadar; wearing white rubber shoes; wielding an umbrella and a battered typewriter, the old man looked as if he should be treading the dusty roads of Mathura (Krishna's birthplace), instead of padding about the mean streets of Manhattan. Was this the man who with only a few rupees in his pockets and no apparent prospects believed that he could travel to America and teach the members of this coarse, materialistic, animal-eating society how to cook and eat vegetarian food? Was this the man who would create Vaishnava temples and vegetarian restaurants in every major city of the world? Was this the man who would establish the first Eastern religion on Western soil since the days of the Roman Empire (the like-

lihood of which theologian Harvey Cox put at one in a million)? Yes, this was he, the dhoti-clad savior that the Western world had been pining for since the death of Pythagoras and Porphyry. This is the man who would teach them not to kill and eat animals, but to eat the prasadam of Lord Krishna."
> —from *Famous Vegetarians* by Rynn Berry

In the 1970s, Bhaktivedanta Swami Prabhupada started a charity program called ISKCON Food Relief [later: "Food for Life"] to feed the poor in India and other parts of the planet.

PAKORAS: VEGETABLE FRITTERS

In India, *pakoras* are almost a national passion. Anywhere people congregate—from bustling city street corners to remote village railway stations—it is a common sight to see a small crowd encircling a hand-pushed *pakora* cart. In snack houses, they are favorites with little more than soup or a beverage. And in the home, from late breakfast to late supper, they are simple, inexpensive, easy-to-make finger foods for drop-in company or a relaxing family break.

Whether you make the fried fritters with vegetables, *panir* cheese or even fruits, there are two methods to choose from: batter-dipped or spoon-fried. The vegetables or other ingredients can simply be cut into rounds, sticks, fan shapes or slices, dipped in seasoned chickpea flour batter and deep-fried, or they can be coarsely chopped or shredded, mixed into a thick batter and spooned into hot oil. Either way, *pakoras* are served piping hot.

There is a choice of batter consistency as well, though the basic principle is to make a texture thick enough to envelop the foods in a thorough coating. A thin batter is used to put a crisp, delicate coating on irregularly-shaped items such as spinach leaves, watercress or Swiss chard leaves. A thick batter is recommended for coating moist foods such as tomatoes or *panir* cheese. A medium-consistency batter will do for such items as eggplant, bell peppers, zucchini, potatoes, blanched cauliflower flowerets and countless more. If you prefer a noticeably crisp outside crust, a little *ghee* or oil is added to the batter and the *pakoras* are fried at a temperature slightly lower than usual, sometimes even double-fried.

CAULIFLOWER PAKORA

Preparation and resting time (after assembling ingredients): 40 minutes. Cooking time: about 30 minutes. Makes: 25-35 pieces

1 1/3 cups sifted chickpea flour (sifted before measuring)
1 tsp salt
2 tsp melted ghee or vegetable oil
2-4 hot green chilies, seeded and minced
1 inch piece of scraped, finely shredded or minced fresh ginger root
1 tsp dry-roasted fenugreek seeds or 1 tblsp coriander seeds

2 tbs coarsely chopped fresh fenugreek or coriander
9 tbs cold water, or enough to make a medium-consistency batter
1/4-1/2 tsp baking powder
ghee or vegetable oil for deep-frying
25-35 cauliflower flowerets, 1 inches long and inch thick, parboiled or half-steamed

Combine the flour, salt, 2 teaspoons *ghee* or vegetable oil, chilies, ginger, fenugreek or coriander seeds, fresh herbs and 7 tablespoons of cold water in a blender or a food processor fitted with the metal blade. Cover and process until smooth. (If you mix the batter by hand, substitute ground spices for the seeds and work with a balloon whisk until smooth.) Gradually add the remaining water, or enough to make a batter the consistency of heavy cream. Cover and set aside for 10-15 minutes.

Again beat with an electric beater, wire whisk or your hand for 2-3 minutes to further lighten the batter. (Check the batter consistency: if it is too thin, moist foods will spatter as they fry; if it is too thick, they will not cook properly. Add flour or water as necessary.) Stir in the baking powder.

Heat 2 1/2 -3 inches of fresh ghee or vegetable oil in a *karai,* wok or deep-frying vessel until the temperature reaches 355°F (180°C). Dip 5 or 6 flowerets in the batter and, one at a time, carefully slip them into the hot oil. The temperature will fall but should then be maintained at between 345°-355°F (173°-180°C) throughout the frying.

Fry until the *pakoras* are golden brown, turning to brown evenly. Remove with a slotted spoon and drain on paper towels. Serve immediately, or keep warm, uncovered, in a preheated 250°F (120°C) oven until all of the *pakoras* are fried, for up to 1/2 hour.

NOTE: It is convenient to keep a bowl of water and tea towels near the frying area. After batter-dipping the items to be fried, rinse and dry your hands before continuing your frying.

—from *Lord Krishna's Cuisine, The Art of Vegetarian Cooking* by Yamuna Devi

---

Edware Espe Brown

Internationally known chef and author of *The Tassajara Bread Book, Tassajara Cooking* and *The Tassajara Recipe Book.*

LENTIL SOUP WITH CUMIN, CORIANDER AND LEMON ZEST

1 cup lentils	1 large carrot, diced
8 cup water	1 tsp freshly ground coriander
bay leaf	1 tsp freshly ground cumin
1 medium yellow onion, diced	zest of 1/2 lemon, minced
2 cloves garlic, minced	salt
2 stalks celery, diced	

Sort through lentils for stones or other debris. Combine in soup pot with water and bay leaf. Bring to boil. Reduce heat, cover and simmer 30 to 45 minutes until lentils are tender. Add onion, garlic, celery and carrot. Continue cooking 30 to 40 minutes until vegetables are tender. Stir in coriander, cumin and lemon zest. Season to taste with salt. Serve hot. Makes 4 to 6 servings.

Lord Buddha

"If there was no one eating meat, then no killing would happen. So eating meat and killing living beings are of the same sin."

—Lord Buddha, from the *Lankavatara Sutra*

MUNG BEANS AND RICE

1 cup mung beans	1 stick cinnamon
5 cups water	1 tsp turmeric
1 cup basmati rice	1 tsp cayenne pepper
2 cups water	1 tsp garam masala
2 tbs sesame seed oil	2 tsp salt
1 tsp black mustard seed	3 tbs grated or chopped
1 tsp cumin seed	ginger (fresh)
3 cloves	

Sauté vegetables (optional: try chopped onions, carrots, zucchini and broccoli fried in sesame oil and 1 tbs. finely chopped ginger).

Rinse, pick over, and boil the mung beans in five cups of water in a heavy skillet. While the mung beans are cooking, soak the rice in 2 cups of water for one-half hour and set aside. In a saucepan sauté the mustard seed, cumin seed, stick cinnamon, and cloves in sesame seed oil. When the mustard seed sputters, lower flame and add the turmeric, cayenne pepper, salt, garam masala, and ginger. Stew for a few minutes over high flame, then turn the spices into the pot of boiling mung beans. Keep cooking the mung beans until most of the liquids have been absorbed, then add the rice plus 2 cups of water. Bring the water to a boil and mix together the rice and mung beans briskly with a wooden spoon. Lower flame and cook gently until rice is soft and fluffy. For a more substantial dish, add sautéed vegetables to the mung beans and rice, after the latter has cooked. Serves 4-6.

Peter Burwash

Peter Burwash first established his reputation as an international tennis player and one of the world's best coaches. Founder of Peter Burwash International, a successful tennis management firm, he has become a sought-after speaker on the topics of service and leadership, giving presentations to businesses around the world. He is the author of four books on tennis, fitness and nutrition. He is a vegetarian since 1970.

NUT LOAF

2 tbs butter or oil
2 stalks celery, chopped
1 carrot, grated
1 cup chopped walnuts
1 cup chopped cashews
1/2 cup ground peanuts
1/4 cup ground sunflower
    seeds

1/2 cup rolled oats
1 pound cottage cheese
1 block tofu, well drained and
    mashed
1/2 tsp basil
1/2 tsp oregano
egg substitute to equal 2 eggs

Lightly sauté the celery in the butter or oil. Mix all ingredients together. Put into a greased 5" x 9" loaf pan and bake for approximately 1 1/2 hours at 375°. Serve hot with gravy or mushroom sauce. Leftovers are great in sandwiches.

—Vegetarian Athletes—

Dave Scott: Only man to win Ironman Triathlon more than twice (six-time winner).

Sixto Linares: World record, 24-hour triathlon (swim 4.8 miles, cycle 185 miles, run 52.5 miles).

Paavo Nurmi: 20 World records in distance running, nine Olympic medals.

Robert Sweetgall: World's premier ultra-distance walker.

Murray Rose: World records, 400 and 1500 meter freestyle.

James and Jonathan de Donato: World records, distance butterfly, stroke swimming.

Bill Pickering: World record, swimming the English Channel.

Estelle Gray and Cheryl Marek: World record, cross-country tandem cycling.

Henry Aaron: All-time major league baseball home run champion.

Robert Parish: Starting center for Boston Celtics, at age 36, 7 ft., 240 lb.

Stan Price: World record, bench press.

Andres Cahling: Mr. International body building champion.

Roy Hilligan: Mr. America body building champion.

Ridgely Abele: 8 National Championships in Karate Association World Championship.
Dan Millman: World Champion gymnast.
Carl Lewis: Winner of nine Olympic gold medals.

[We obtained this information from EarthSave Foundation, 706 Frederick Street, Santa Cruz, California 95062-2205.]

Caitanya Mahaprabhu

Sri Caitanya appeared 500 years ago in West Bengal, India, and became the pioneer of a great social and religious movement in India. He inaugurated and masterminded the first mass nonviolent civil disobedience resistance and a spiritual revolution directed inward, toward a scientific understanding of the highest knowledge of the human spiritual nature. Considered an Avatar of Lord Krishna, he resided for the last 20 years of his life in Puri, Orissa.

Sri Caitanya used to daily visit the temple of Lord Jagannatha in Puri. Every year, in the summer, the main attraction of this holy place, the Festival of the Chariots, honors Lord Jagannatha as Lord of the Universe. The celebration draws millions of pilgrims from across the subcontinent and has been held in Puri for the past two thousand years.

The temple of Jagannath is one of the most famous of all India and is known for its spiritual food, *prasad,* that is distributed every day to thousands of pilgrims. The Festival of the Chariots, since the Sixties, has been brought to all the major cities of the world by the members of the International Society for Krishna Consciousness.

BUNCHI MOONG DAL KICHARI
LAVISH RICE AND MUNG

Preparation and cooking time (after assembling ingredients): 1 1/4 hours. Serves: 6

1 cup (95 g) basmati or other long-grain white rice
3/4 cup (170 g) split moong

dal, without skins, sorted, washed and drained
1 1/2 tsp (7 ml) turmeric
about 8 cups (2 liters) water

1/2 cup (120 ml) ghee or a
mixture of vegetable oil and
unsalted butter
1/3 cup (45 g) raw cashew bits
or halves
1/3 cup (40 g) sliced raw
almonds
1/4 cup (25 g) fresh or dried
ribbon coconut
1/3 cup (45 g) raisins or
currants
3-inch (7.5 cm) piece of cinnamon stick
8 whole cloves
1 tbs. (15 ml) cumin seeds
1-2 whole dried red chilies

2 tbs (30 ml) raw sugar or
equivalent sweetener
1/4 tsp (1 ml) yellow asafetida
powder (hing) (This amount
applies only to yellow
Cobra brand. Reduce any
other asafetida by three-
fourths.)
1 cup (240) fresh green peas
or frozen baby peas,
defrosted
2 1/2 - 3 tsps (12-15 ml) salt
2 tbs (30 ml) butter or ghee
3 tbs (45 ml) minced fresh
parsley or coarsely chopped
coriander

If basmati rice is used, clean, wash, soak and drain. Combine the split moong dal, rice and turmeric in a bowl, sprinkle in about 1 tsp. (5 ml) of the water and stir until the mixture is coated with the turmeric.

Heat the ghee or oil-butter mixture in a heavy 3-4 quart/liter nonstick saucepan over moderate heat. One after another, separately fry the cashew nuts, almonds and coconut, until they each become golden brown. As the batches brown, remove with a slotted spoon and transfer to paper towels to drain. Add the raisins and mix well. Increase the heat to moderately high, add the cinnamon stick, cloves, cumin seeds, red chilies and sweetener and fry until the cumin seeds darken and the sweetener caramelizes and turns a rich reddish-brown.

—from *Lord Krishna's Cuisine* by Yamuna Devi, Bala Books

━━━━━━━━━

Greg Caton is president of Lumen Foods and a world leader in the manufacture of meat analogs, soy protein specialties and high protein snacks. Lumen Foods, 409 Scott Street, Lake Charles, LA 70601, USA. (318) 436-6748, fax (318) 436-1769, order line (800) 256-2253

"Men have held vegetarians to a small minority in our most

advanced society. Why? I believe it has been habit. In all ways men are creatures of habit. As George Bernard Shaw once said, 'There is no abomination which custom will not legitimate.' When I discovered that I was in a position to advance the development of meat substitutes through a simple processing technique that had not yet been commercialized, I saw the ultimate solution to making vegetarianism a mainstream practice. And history was on my side: in 1945 a little known vegetable product was being distributed to replace an animal food, butter. Most people thought it was a fad, a joke, made available only because the war effort was making butter a rationed commodity. But by 1958 margarine had replaced butter as the world's most popular edible fat. A complete change in people's dietary habit. All in one generation. I wanted to do to meat what margarine had done to butter. I saw an opportunity in my own lifetime to bring to fruition the prediction of Leonardo da Vinci: 'The time will come when men such as I will look on the murder of animals as they now look on the murder of men.'

"What will make this possible is a change in our habits. And this is simply because men cannot embrace an ethical or moral concept, however self-evident, if they are not able to modify their behavior to employ it. Meat substitutes will supply the missing key. Once people are able to so easily change their habits, they will accept the self evident. I have seen the future and it is vegetarian…but the road to get there is lined with substitutes."

—Greg Caton

Lumen is the term Greg Caton is using to describe a whole range of products that have the "look, taste and texture" of real meat products—a meat replacer that doesn't require refrigeration, is easy to use, easy to store, comes in numerous flavors and can be used in almost any recipe calling for real meat.

VEGETARIAN CHICKEN SALAD

Heartline Chicken Fillet (reconstituted)

To reconstitute Heartline Meatless Meats, add 3/4 cup of water to each cup of "meat"—(enough water to completely cover). Bring to a boil and cover. Cook for 10 minutes, or more to desired texture (not letting it run out of water).

Diced onions	**Mayonnaise (or mayo**
Diced celery	**substitute)**
Pickle relish	

Cool reconstituted Chicken Fillet. Chop or put through food grinder or food processor. Add dices onions, dices celery, pickle relish and mayonnaise to taste. Suggestions: Serve on crackers, sandwiches or salad.

───────────

Lee Chamberlin, actress

PASTA ARAME WITH OYSTER MUSHROOMS

Arame is a delicate tasting seaweed. It can be found dried. Most health food stores carry this sea vegetable in packets. Oyster Mushrooms can be found dried or fresh. Fresh is recommended for flavor as well as nutritional value. Tamari Sauce, a fermented soybean mash, is lighter in taste and consistency than the average soy sauce.

1 cup dry arame	**2 cloves freshly crushed garlic**
12 to 18 whole oyster mush-	**1 small red bell pepper**
** rooms**	**8 oz. package thin spaghetti or**
1-2 tbs tamari sauce	** angel hair pasta**
1-2 tbs olive oil	**kelp (optional)**

Slice red bell pepper into thin strips. Place in pan of water, enough to cover bottom of the pan, cover and steam lightly. Pepper should remain relatively crisp, not mushy. Drain on a towel and set aside. Rinse the arame in a colander, place in a pan with enough water to cover the arame.

Simmer covered for 10 to 15 minutes until soft but not mushy. Season lightly with 1-2 tbs. of tamari (too much tamari can impose too strong a soy flavor, so taste test).

Remove arame from pan and set aside. Lightly sauté mushroom in enough olive oil to coat the pan. Mushrooms should not be cooked as much as slightly softened. Place softened mushrooms on a paper towel to drain. Add a touch more olive oil to the pan if needed and sauté the garlic. Leave the garlic in the pan.

Cook pasta according to package directions, drain in a colander. (If desired, shake a modest amount of kelp onto the pasta. Be aware that too much kelp combined with the arame and the tamari might result in saltiness, so use your judgment and your taste buds.)

Heat olive oil and garlic, add mushrooms and warm both ingredients. Make a bed of your pasta, pour olive oil, mushroom and garlic over it. Sprinkle arame, which is black in color, over the pasta, add the thin slices of red bell pepper around and on top of the arame and pasta for a dish both pleasing to the eye and the tongue.

━━━━━━━━━━

Deen B. Chandora, M.D. is a renowned Internist, Psychiatrist, Addiction Medicine Specialist and Diplomat of Forensic Medicine. He has presented many research papers in Gastroenterology, Internal Medicine, Psychiatry, Cultural Anthropology and Religion. He studied nutrition while doing residency in Internal Medicine. He is a trustee and founder of Vedic Temple, Atlanta. Currently he is a Medical Director of Clayton Mental Health Center, Georgia, USA.

COCONUT BURFI

4 cups milk	**1/3 cup shredded or flaked**
1/2 cup heavy cream	**coconut (unsweetened)**
1 cup turbinado sugar	**1 tsp vanilla**

In large heavy saucepan (preferably nonstick) put milk and cream. Bring to a boil over medium-high heat, stirring occasionally to prevent sticking. Stirring often and scraping the bottom of the saucepan, keep the milk boiling (but reduce the heat if the milk starts to boil over). The milk will begin to thicken after approximately 1/2 hour. When the boiling action slows to a cooking, stir constantly until a small amount of the mixture dropped into very cold water forms a small soft ball.

Stir in coconut and cook just 3 minutes longer.

Empty burfi onto a flat, buttered tray and mold into a square 1/2 inch thick. Cool at room temperature. Cut into desired portions. This burfi can be made up to 2 days in advance of serving, but must be refrigerated. Remove from refrigerator 1 hour before serving.

━━━━━━━━━━

Terry Cole-Whittaker is author of *What You Think of Me Is None of My Business*, a yogini and spiritual teacher.

SUNFLOWER SEED CHEESE

2 cups hulled sunflower seeds soaked in water for 12 hours then drained. Rinse two times a day for one or two days.

Place sprouted sunflower seeds in food processor with the juice of one and half or two lemons, add one quarter of a cup of olive oil or flax oil, one tablespoon asafetida or garlic to taste, add one tablespoon Braggs aminos or salt to taste and blend. If too dry, add a little water. Serve with bread, crackers or chips. Everyone loves this food. It is healthy and delicious.

━━━━━━━━━━

Michael Cremo is co-author of *Forbidden Archeology: The Hidden History of the Human Race*, Torchlight Publishing and *Divine Nature,* Bhaktivedanta Book Trust.

MANGO DESSERT

3 ripe mangos (peeled and pitted)
15-ounce can sweetened condensed milk
juice from 1 lemon

1 cup raspberries (fresh or frozen)
1/4 cup orange juice
4 tablespoons chopped pistachio nuts

Marinate raspberries in orange juice. Place mangos, sweetened condensed milk, and lemon juice in a blender. Blend until smooth. Pour half of this mixture evenly into 4 dessert dishes. Divide 3/4 cup raspberries evenly into the dishes, then add the remainder of the mango mixture.

Chill for several hours. Immediately before serving, top with remaining berries and garnish with pistachio nuts. Serves 4.

Alfred Ford

"I became a part-time vegetarian when I was in college. It just seemed disgusting to me to consume carcasses of dead animals. When I joined the Hare Krishnas in 1974, my diet became strictly vegetarian. My great-grandfather, Henry Ford, was also interested in vegetarianism. He was influenced by the Seventh Day Adventist Western Health Reform Institute, founded in Battle Creek, Michigan in 1866. One of their dire warnings was about putrefaction of meat in the stomach. Henry Ford 'came to see the body as another sort of machine whose efficiency depended on the type of fuel fed its boiler.' (quoted from Robert Lacey's *Ford, The Men And The Machine*, Little Brown 1986)

"My great-grandfather was especially interested in the use of soya beans. He was the first person to become involved in growing and harvesting soya beans on a major scale. He even used them in the manufacture of his automobiles! In our home we tend more towards the soya bean product, tofu, flavoring it with some Indian spices in a kind of East-meets-West recipe. Henry Ford's commitment to soya bean research has produced many healthful and delicious products, essential to today's vegetarian diet."

SPICY SAUTÉED TOFU

Take one block of tofu and chop up into small cubes. Take 2 tbs. of olive oil and bring to high heat in a heavy-based skillet. Add a half teaspoon of hing (asafetida) and a quarter teaspoon of cayenne and lightly brown them. Mix in the cut-up tofu with a half teaspoon of turmeric. Sauté by stirring frequently with a spatula for 20-30 minutes.

=====

Dr. Michael Fox

America's leading veterinarian, vice-president of The Humane Society of the United States and Director, Center for Respect of Life and Environment in Washington, D.C. Also, syndicated columnist and author of more than 30 books, most recently *Inhumane Society: The American Way of Animal Exploitation* and *You Can Save the Animals, 50 Things to Do Right Now*, printed by St. Martin's Press, 175 Fifth Avenue, New York, NY 10010.

Fox is an internationally known defender of the animal kingdom. He travels widely, lecturing on animal behavior, conservation, animal rights, humane and sustainable agriculture, and a creation-centered spirituality.

BASIC VEGAN CURRY CASSEROLE

Preheat oven to 300°. Dice 1 onion and 2 garlic cloves (and 1/2 green pepper and add pinch of cumin seeds). Sauté onion and garlic in 3 tbs.. vegetable oil. Add 1 tbs. of curry powder when onion is half-cooked. Stir. Chop fresh raw vegetables* of your choice (potato, peas, green beans, cauliflower, broccoli, etc.) and steam until half-cooked.

Stir onion-curry mix with steamed vegetables in a casserole dish (lightly greased with vegetable oil) and add 1 can stewed tomatoes or small can tomato paste.** Bake at 300° until vegetables are cooked just right. Serve on a bed of rice with sweet chutney and chapatis.***

*Experiment with different vegetables: add sesame seeds, chick peas, lentils or cashew nuts; mix in some tofu cut in cubes.

**Substituite 1 cube vegetable bullion and 1 tbs. miso ≐ 1 cup water = 1/2 lime(juice) for tomato paste for a change, or 2 T. peanut butter.

*** Making chapatis is easy. Prepare a dough of half whole wheat and half white flour, roll into round pieces 1/4" thick, 8" across and dry-fry (no oil) in a flat skillet at medium to medium-high heat.

Animal Bill of Rights
from *You Can Save the Animals* by Michael Fox

- Animals have the right to equal and fair consideration and to be treated with humane concern and responsibility.
- Animals have the right to live free from human exploitation, whether in the name of science or sport, exhibition or service, food or fashion.
- Animals have the right to live in harmony with their nature, rather than in accordance with human desires.
- Animals have the right to live on a healthy planet.
- Endangered species have the right to life and habitat preservation.
- Animals have the right to be protected from physical or mental suffering when subject to any form of human exploitation .
- Domestic animals have the right to live in adequate physical and social environment.
- Animals have the right to be regarded as "ours" only in sacred trust.

"In most restaurants, vegetable soup contains chicken stock, and baked goods contain eggs and dairy products. The film and phonograph records we buy include gelatins and other slaughterhouse by-products, as does our bone china. Most protein-enriched shampoos and skin creams contain animal by-products and even fetal fluids and glandular extracts. Soap sometimes contains the tallow not only of exhausted dairy cows and over-fattened chickens, pigs, and cattle, but also of the estimated 7.5 million cats and dogs that are exterminated each year in animal shelters across the United States."
—from *Cruelty-Free Living* by Dr. Michael W. Fox, published in *The Green Lifestyle Handbook*, edited by Jeremy Rifkin and published by Henry Holt & Company/NY.

Saint Francis of Assisi
"Praise be to thee, O Lord, for our Mother the Earth, who sustains and nourishes us, bringing forth diverse fruits and flowers of many colors, and the grass."

Vegetarian Catholics refer often to the inspiring example set by St. Francis of Assisi, the patron saint of animals, always caring for the well-being of all the creatures of God.

This very old and simple recipe was given to us by Luciana Trionfetti, known in the Assisi area as a dynamic promoter of vegetarianism and animal rights.

FRANCISCAN CHICKPEAS

chickpeas	olive oil extra virgin
1 clove garlic	salt
1 or more branches of fresh rosemary	

Soak the chickpeas in water for 15 hours. Then boil them in abundant water, slightly salted, till the chickpeas are tender and mash easily (usually takes around 30 minutes). In a casserole fry in olive oil, the garlic and the rosemary (this ingredient can be wrapped in a thin cheesecloth to get its flavor without it losing its leaves in the preparation) till the garlic assumes a golden color. Then pour in the drained chickpeas and let them fry a little. Add some of the salted water you cooked the chickpeas in—enough to cover the peas—and let cook on a low flame till some of the water is evaporated. Mash one fourth of the chickpeas into a puree and then mix it with the rest, remove the rosemary and savor with olive oil.

Phil Gallelli

Phil Gallelli is the publisher and co-founder of Bala Books. He has been a vegetarian since the age of 14. As an internationally acclaimed publisher of children's classics and award winning alternative life style publications, he has produced some significant works on vegetarianism. One of his most recognized publishing efforts was the critically acclaimed cookbook, *Lord Krishna's Cuisine, The Art of Indian Vegetarian Cooking*, by Yamuna Devi. This was the first non-Western cuisine cookbook to ever receive the prestigious IACP award, being hailed as the BOOK OF THE YEAR, in 1987. He has also published academic works on vegetarianism such as Steven Rosen's *Food for the Spirit, Vegetarianism and the World Religions* with a preface by Nobel laureate Isaac Bashevis Singer. He resides in southern California with his wife and their five children. The following recipe submitted by his wife, Lory Gallelli, was a family favorite in her native country of Italy.

EGGPLANT SPREAD

1 large ripe eggplant, peeled
and cubed
2 cups sun dried tomatoes
1 cup capers
1 cup black olives
3 tbs olive oil

1 cup chopped onions
5 cloves garlic, crushed
10 fresh basil leaves
1 tbs salt
1/2 tsp black pepper

Sauté in olive oil, onion, garlic and basil in a large skillet until the onions are clear. Add eggplant salt and pepper, cover and let mixture cook slowly for 45 minutes. When the eggplant mixture has cooked, combine with tomatoes and olives and puree, Serve warm with your favorite breads.

Mahatma Gandhi

This is the bread of the Indians. Gandhi used to eat daily rice, chapatis and vegetables.

CHAPATIS

1 cup fine whole wheat flour   1/2-1/4 cup warm water

Knead water into flour until a pliable dough forms. Divide dough into 6 balls. Heat frying pan. On a floured surface, roll each ball into a thin round. Place chapati on heated pan. When bubbles appear, bake briefly on other side. Using tongs, place chapati directly over open flame until it puffs up. Flip back and forth until speckled brown. Spread with ghee or butter. Yields 6 chapatis.

Quotes from Mahatma Gandhi
(1869-1948)

Civilized Society

"I do feel that spiritual progress does demand at some stage that we should cease to kill our fellow creatures for the satisfaction of our bodily wants."

"The greatness of a nation and its moral progress can be judged by the way its animal are treated."

Holy Cow

"The cow is a poem of compassion…to protect her is to protect all the creatures of God's creation."

Adopt A Little Humility

"What I want to bring to your notice is that vegetarians need to be tolerant if they want to convert others to vegetarianism. Adopt a little humility. We should appeal to the moral sense of the people who do not see eye to eye with us. If a vegetarian became ill and took a doctor's prescription for beef tea, then I would not call him a vegetarian. A vegetarian is made of sterner stuff. Why? Because it is the building of the spirit and not of the body. Man is more than meat. It is the spirit in man with which we are concerned. Therefore, vegetarians should have that moral basis that a man was not born a carnivorous animal, but born to live on the fruits and herbs that the Earth grows."

Maneka Gandhi

She was twice Minister of State for Environment & Forests in the Indian Cabinet. She worked for radical reforms to protect the environment and create sustainable development alternatives. A renowned animal rights activist, she is the founder of People for Animals, 510 Prasad Chambers, Opera House, Bombay 400-004, India.

Our Vegetarian Bodies

"The human body is designed to be vegetarian. Our tooth structure is vegetarian—with small canines and powerful molars. Our enzymes for digestion are designed to digest vegetarian food rather than meat. But most important our intestines are specifically designed only for vegetarian food. The carnivorous animal intestine is designed by both its smooth stovepipe shape and short length to have short transit times. Short, straight chutes—in and out. We have an enormously long 26-foot intestine—like all grass eating animals—convoluted and winding like mountain roads with deeply grooved bowel walls, full of pouches.

"What happens when you eat meat? A meat eater must produce extensive bile acids in his stomach to digest his meat, specially deoxycholic acid. This acid is converted by the clostridia bacteria in the meat eater's intestine into powerful carcinogens. Meat takes so long to go round and round the intestine that they rot inside turning toxic."
—from *Heads & Tails* by Maneka Gandhi,
The People For Animals Edition

BAGHARE BAINGAM

This is a common dish in India and each household has its own variation of the stuffing of the brinjal (eggplant).
Preparation time: 30 minutes. Cooking time: 1 hour. Serves 6-8 persons

1/2 kg brinjals small and round
25 gms coconut grated and roasted dry
6 gms sesame seeds roasted dry
3 gms cumin seeds roasted
12 gms roasted peanuts
1 tbs. fresh coriander leaves
15 gms red chilies, powdered and roasted dry
3 gms coriander seeds powdered and roasted dry
6 gms ginger scraped and ground
6 gms garlic ground
6 gms parched grams powdered
1 1/2 gm garam masala powder (a powdered mixture of cloves, cardamom and cinnamon)
115 gms onion finally chopped
12 gm tamarind pulp

Slit brinjal in fours leaving the stem intact. The brinjals should be whole with deep cuts.

Soak tamarind in a cup of warm water for a while. Strain and keep aside. Grind finely together coconut, sesame seeds, cumin seeds, molasses, peanuts and coriander leaves with little water. Add salt, red chilies, coriander seeds, turmeric, ginger, garlic, parched grams and garam masala powder. Mix well. Fill this into the brinjals. If the stuffing is in excess, spread it over the brinjals while cooking. Heat the oil. When smoking hot, remove from fire and cool a bit. Put back on fire.

Fry the brinjals lightly, 3-4 at time. Keep aside. In the same oil fry the chopped onion to a light golden color. Add brinjals and tamarind juice. Cover and cook on low heat. Stir occasionally, taking care not to break the brinjals.

When cooked, dry the liquid completely.

Boy George
"I do believe that as long as we are slaughtering animals we will also be slaughtered. Like George Bernard Shaw said, 'Cruelty begets its offspring, war.'"
> —from his autobiography, *Take It Like A Man*,
> Harper Collins

Boy George is a strong promoter of vegetarianism and speaks often to other rock stars about his choice, which he considers spiritual. Speaking about a friend he wrote, "John Richardson, who used to be the drummer in the Seventies glam group The Rubettes, is the best advertisement for vegetarianism and spiritual life. Even my most cynical friends have taken to him. He and his family have always shown me total warmth and his wife Satchi makes killer *Prasadam*."

Prasadam means mercy and is the name of the pure vegetarian food cooked and offered with love to Krishna, God, according to the ancient traditions of the Vedas.

SEITAN STIR FRIES

Seitan (wheat gluten)	**Tamari sauce**
Garlic	**Ginger**

Onions

Sliced burdock root

Chili powder

Olive oil (extra virgin cold
    pressed)

Almond milk cheese

Slice 1 1/2 inch pieces of seitan. Stir fry with olive oil and tamari
sauce on low flame, use heavy iron fry pan or until all the oil and
tamari are absorbed and seitan crispy. Take out seitan (keep juices),
add veggies and stir fry in olive oil with ginger, garlic, chili powder
and salt to taste. Mix in the seitan, throw in the pan scrapings. Top
with layer of almond cheese, put under broiler or oven for 5 minutes
until cheese melts and turns brown. Serves 4

=====

Arthur Goldberg
    Vegetarian leader and publisher of *Veggie Single News*
[Helping Vegetarians (and those who want to be) Meet & Eat]
P.O. Box 300412, Brooklyn, NY 11230-0412, USA,
(718) 437-0190, fax (718) 633-9817

The magazine began as *Vegetarian Single News*. Explains Arthur
Goldberg: "Our goal for the publication has expanded too. In the
beginning, I saw my job as simply creating a magazine that helps individual vegetarian singles meet and connect. I now realize that our
efforts have a much more important ultimate purpose. We have, without originally being aware of it, become an important instrument for
tying together and strengthening the vegetarian community nationwide....Our personal ads allow and encourage veggies (and veggie
hopefuls) to meet each other locally or far away and share time,
conversation and when the chemistry is right, intimacy.
    "In short, while the content of our magazine need not change,
our purpose is now two-fold. We are here not only to help individual
veggies but to help build the vegetarian community and the vegetarian movement."

Questions from Carnivores by Arthur Goldberg

Q: In nature animals kill and eat other animals. So how can it be
wrong for people to eat animals too?

A: In nature, animals often eat other animals while they are still alive. Animals sometimes rape each other, steal each other's food and homes and kill each other's children. Do you really base your ethics on what animals do? The animals that we choose to eat are not carnivores anyway. We tend to pick up peaceful, gentle domesticated animals like cows, lambs and rabbits to kill for food, partly because they are more easily controlled. In addition, modern factory farming doesn't just slaughter the animals. It involves their absolute enslavement from birth, the removal of their children at tender young ages and the total denial of each being's physical, social and psychological needs. They are usually chained up in a dark solitary pen in the interest of creating the most meat in the shortest time as cheaply as possible. This lifelong torture, for purposes of profit, culminates in an impersonal assembly-line death handled by machines. The animals are not just simply killed as by predators.

Q: If you don't eat meat, fish or poultry, then you have to kill and eat plants. Isn't that just as bad as killing animals? (The person asking this is not really interested in the welfare of plants. It is a trick question meant to catch you off guard.)

A: Plants do not have the complex nervous systems of animals. For that reason, as well as common observation, there is little evidence that plants suffer or experience pain or anxiety. Animals, on the other hand, feel pain every bit as much as human beings and may even suffer more because they don't understand what is happening to them. If you are truly interested in saving plants, you would still eat vegetarian. To create meat, an animal must consume many times his own weight in plants. It has been estimated that the inefficiencies of meat production are such that each pound of meat results in the destruction of at least 10 pounds of plants. Therefore, a human will kill many less plants by eating them directly than by eating animals raised on plants.

Eggplant Casserole

3 tbs soy butter or oil
1 onion chopped (I like large chunks or slices)
3-4 ribs celery chopped
1 green pepper chopped

1/2 cup canned or 1-2 skinned fresh tomatoes, chopped
1/2 cup water
1 medium eggplant (1 lb.)
6 oz. sliced fresh mushrooms may be added

1 tsp. basil
1 tbs. parsley (optional)
1 tsp. oregano

salt and pepper to taste
3 slices whole wheat bread
egg substitute (equivalent to
two eggs)

Preheat oven to 325 degrees. Soak bread in water. Sauté onion and celery. Add all seasonings and vegetables. Mix. Simmer just until tender
(not too long). Squeeze out excess water from bread. Mix bread with
egg substitute. Combine egg bread and vegetable mixture. Place in
oiled baking dish. Bake covered 25 minutes and uncovered 10-15 minutes. Makes about 4-5 servings.

Dick Gregory
From *The New Vegetarians* by Rynn Berry, Pythagorean
Publishers, PO Box 8174, JAF Station, New York, NY 10116:

Q. Is your family vegetarian as well?
A. Yes, my whole family is vegetarian. Ten of my eleven kids fast one
day a week, and there hasn't been so much as one runny nose among
them.
Q. Have you influenced members of the black community to become
vegetarian? Are a lot of black people becoming vegetarian now?
A. Oh yes, it's just unbelievable, unbelievable. I would say that I am
one of the biggest influences in America today on both blacks and
whites, mainly because of my college appearances. And in every book
I write, I always mention something about vegetarianism.
Q. I read that you ran 900 miles, taking only a kelp-based liquid formula as nourishment.
A. It was a formula called "4-X". It had about 17 different ingredients:
kelp was the major ingredient. This formula could feed about 2 billion
people a day, 3 meals a day for 32 cents, at a manufactured cost of a
nickel.

The following recipe is from *Dick Gregory's Natural Diet for
Folks Who Eat: Cooking with Mother Nature*, Harper and Row.

MIXED SALAD

Mix well: shredded cabbage, grated cabbage and chopped minced or grated onions.
Garnish with pumpkin, sunflower or sesame seeds.
Top with a salad dressing.

French dressing: Combine 1/2 cup of olive oil, 1/4 cup lemon juice, the juice of 1 tomato or 1/4 cup lemon juice (freshly squeezed). Mix all ingredients thoroughly (use blender if available).

George Harrison

George became vegetarian when he was introduced with the other Beatles to the transcendental meditation of Maharishi Mahesh Yogi. More than any other member of the famous group, through his music he made vegetarianism, yoga and Indian philosophy very popular among the youth of the late 60s. Some of his songs—"Here Comes the Sun", "Within You, Without You", "While My Guitar Gently Weeps", "My Sweet Lord"—have become rock 'n' roll classics.

DARK HORSE LENTIL SOUP

1 red chili
1 tsp. cumin seeds
2 large onions, chopped
2 cloves garlic
1 cup lentils (one or more
   types of lentils can be used)

2 large tomatoes, chopped
2 green peppers, chopped
1 bay leaf
Salt and pepper to taste

Heat a small amount of oil in a frying pan. When oil is good and hot add the red chili and cumin seeds. When the seeds stop sputtering, brown the onions and garlic in seasoned oil. In a separate deep pan, wash the lentils in plenty of water. When clean, liberally cover with water.

When the onions are browned, add them to the pan of lentils. Now add the tomatoes, peppers, bay leaf, salt and pepper. Potatoes and carrots and small boiling onions may be added for a more substantial meal. Bring to a boil, cover and turn down to a very low heat. The soup is ready to serve in an hour and tastes even better the next day. Serves 4.

—'Dark Horse Lentil Soup' from
Mary Frampton and Friends, Rock and Roll Recipes by Mary Frampton. Reprinted by permission of Doubleday & Company.

James Higgins, astrologer

ASTRO BURGER

2 cups of brown rice or instant brown rice if you are in a hurry; cook the rice and let it sit for 15 minutes
3 tsp of peanut butter
1/2 tsp salt

1 tsp. of basil
1/2 tsp. ground cumin
1 12 oz tub tofu (regular not soft)
1/4 tsp. black pepper or 1/8 tsp. cayenne pepper

Mix all the ingredients together in a mixing bowl, then you butter a frying pan or a skillet and then make the mixture into hamburger style patties. Fry them on the pan or skillet for 12 minutes on a medium heat, until they look brown; then you flip them over.

If you like, slice some cheese on top. Cook another ten minutes, put the burger on a bun and add lettuce, tomatoes, onions, ketchup and mustard.

American Fast Food

The demand for beef by American fast food restaurants is a major reason for the destruction of Central American rain forests. This contributes to both species extinction and, along with other defor-estation, contributes to carbon dioxide pollution, a major factor in the greenhouse effect. Topsoil depletion, a historic demise of many great civilizations, has reached 75% in the U.S. and 85% of this loss is directly related to livestock production. More than half the water used for all purposes in this country goes to livestock production. As individuals, we can take some comfort in knowing that, with a vegetarian diet, each of us saves one acre of trees each year. That is sort of like having a private forest, even if you live in a high-rise in New York or Chicago.

The Cost of the Burger

Common hamburger would cost $35/lb. if water used by the meat industry were not subsidized by U.S. taxpayers.

Are you one of them?

Are you aware that the American government sustains the meat industry by permitting grazing on public lands, and by offering administrative services, subsidies, insurance and mortgage programs, tax write-offs, price supports and outright grants. Do your legislators know what you think about it? Are you tired of paying the "hidden" cost of meat? Let them know how you feel about this issue.

"We in America are hooked," said Francis Moore Lappé, author of the best-seller *Diet For A Small Planet*, "on gas-guzzling automobiles because of the illusion of cheap petroleum. Likewise, we got hooked on a grain-fed, meat-centered diet because of the illusion of cheap grain."

If the whole world would follow the standard American diet, according to American scientist David Pimentel, the planet's entire petroleum reserves would be exhausted in 13 years.

John Hogue

Philosopher and scholar, he is considered one of the top authorities on Nostradamus. Author of *Nostradamus and the Millennium, The Millennium Book of Prophecy* and *Nostradamus, The New Revelations*, Hogue is a much in demand guest on many radio and TV programs worldwide.

QUINCE JELLY

This recipe is derived from an original recipe of Nostradamus.

Quinces look like apples or pears and have a wonderful scent and aroma. The ancient Greeks imported these fruits from the Eastern Caucasus and cooked them together with honey into a quince butter named Melimelon.

The Romans discovered quinces growing on Crete and named them Cretan Apples (Malum Cidoneum) and planted and grew them in their Northern provinces. The quinces were considered a symbol of fertility and sacred to the goddess of love, Aphrodite.

The Portuguese liked this fruit which they named "marmelo" (from which the name marmalade developed). They planted quinces in abundance and even exported them. Thus, quinces made their way into all of Europe and the rest of the world. Nostradamus wrote that Quince Jelly is a magnificent means to fortify amorous strength and sexual sensitivity and was appreciated by Dukes and Kings. It was prepared and served to King Francis as well to Cardinal of Clermont.

Quinces are ideal for marmalades or jellies because of their high content of pectin. The pear shaped quince has a richer flavor and therefore is widely preferred over the apple shaped quince.

All types of quinces, when cooked, produce a light red juice. To prepare quinces for cooking: simply wash them (brushing off the peach-like velveteen fuzz) and cut into pieces (the seeds do not need to be removed, since they are, when completely cooked, strained through a cheese cloth).

1.500 grams (3 lb. + 10 oz) quinces
1/4 liter (1/2 pint) water
1.800 grams (4 lb.) sugar

5 grams (1/2 teaspoon) lemon acid (optional)
1/2 to 1 pack pectin

After cutting quinces, place them in a pot with water and cook until soft (approximately 35 minutes). Don't let them get mushy. Put a cheesecloth over a bowl, not tight but with a good dent, pour quinces and water into cheesecloth and let it drain overnight. Put quince juice into a large pot and add sugar and bring to a vigorous boil (for about a minute), stir frequently—turn off heat and make gelling test (1 drop on a porcelain or glass plate, place into refrigerator for a few minutes—if it's running, you need to add pectin).

Stir in pectin and bring to a second boil. You do not want it to be so stiff that you have to cut it with a knife; it should have a smooth runny consistency. According to manufacturer's recommendation, put into clean jars and seal it with cellophane wrap. Makes about five to six 1/2 lb. jars.

―――――――

Jesus Christ

According to many Biblical scholars, Jesus Christ was an Essene and it is well attested that the Essenes were devout vegetarians. Their chief article of diet was a loaf of bread made from sprouted wheat.

ESSENE SPROUTED BREAD

1 1/2 cups wheat berries
2 cups water

Soak the wheatberries overnight in a bowl with enough water to cover the berries. Then drain in a colander. Wrap the berries in a tea towel made of cheesecloth or muslin. Store them in a cool dark place to facilitate germination. After three days, hundreds of whiskery shoots will be poking through the holes in the cheesecloth. The berries have started to sprout! Remove the sprouted berries from the cloth and rinse them thoroughly. Don't bother to dry them but place them into a blender with the water still clinging to the sprouts. Puree them for about 2 minutes. This should yield a mushy dough. Add just a bit more water to give the dough a pasty consistency.

Remove from the blender and knead by hand for about 10 minutes until the ball of dough gets softer. (Before kneading it is a good idea to coat one's hands with oil to keep them from getting gummed up with dough.) Hand-shape the dough into a round loaf and place on an oiled baking sheet. Preheat the oven to 350∞F, and bake for about an hour or until the loaf is baked through and browned on top. Serves 4.

―――――――

Dr. John Harvey Kellogg

"How is it that the life of the inventor of America's most quintes-

sential food—peanut butter and cornflakes—is so little known? John Harvey Kellogg was the Edison of the epigastrium, the Einstein of the colon. Not only was he America's most prolific food inventor, but in his heyday, in the latter part of the nineteenth century, he was also the greatest abdominal surgeon in the world. Yet today he is remembered, if at all, because his name adorns the packages of America's best-selling cereals. A firm believer in Hippocrates dictum that 'Our medicine should be our food, and our food should be our medicine.'—Dr. Kellogg held that a low protein diet strengthened resistance to disease, promoted longevity, and increased physical and mental endurance; whereas a high protein diet overtaxed the kidneys and liver, and contributed to the accumulation of toxins in the intestines."
—from *Famous Vegetarians* by Rynn Berry

Kellogg invented cornflakes as an alternative to the traditional American breakfast of bacon 'n' eggs, which he considered to be nutritionally unsound. As a result of his having invented cornflakes, millions of people now enjoy a meatless breakfast of cereal and milk.

ASPARAGUS ON TOAST (WITH SOY CREAM SAUCE)

12 asparagus spears (trimmed and scrubbed)

6 slices whole-wheat toast	**2 tbs flour**
6 pats soy margarine	**1/4 tsp nutmeg**
1 tsp sea salt	**1/2 tsp sea salt**
1 cup boiling water	**1/2 pint soy milk**
	1 cup asparagus cooking
Cream Sauce:	**liquid (obtained by boiling**
2 tbs soy margarine	**asparagus)**

Wash trim and scrub asparagus spears.

In a skillet bring to a boil 1 cup of salted water. Add asparagus spears. As soon as the water resumes boiling, lower heat, cover and let simmer for 5 minutes. Be careful not to overcook! When tender, remove asparagus from the skillet, and drain. Reserve the asparagus cooking liquid for the cream sauce. Spread pats of soy margarine on the toast. Cut the spears into four-inch lengths, and cover the buttered side of the toast slice with asparagus pieces.

Cream Sauce: melt the soy margarine in a saucepan. Stir in the flour, nutmeg and sea salt. Combine the asparagus liquid with the soy milk, and gradually stir into the margarine and flour mixture. Stir over a low flame until mixture thickens. When it reaches a thick, creamy consistency, pour (piping hot) over the asparagus and toast. Serves 4.

Shri Krishna

"If one offers Me with love and devotion a leaf, a flower, fruit, or water, I will accept."

So spoke Krishna in the *Bhagavad-gita* more than 5000 years ago. After presenting to Arjuna various kinds of yoga, Krishna presents *bhakti* (devotional service) as the highest form of yoga. Krishna means All-Attractive and is one of the names of God.

"Of all yogis, one who always abides in Me with great faith, worshipping Me in transcendental loving service, is most intimately united with Me in yoga and is highest of all."

Summarizing the process of *bhakti-yoga,* the yoga of devotion, Lord Krishna says: "All that you do, all that you eat, all that you offer and give away, should be done as an offering unto Me.'"

The Yoga of Eating

All the different yoga systems promote a pure vegetarian diet. Offering vegetarian food is an integral part of *bhakti,* the yoga of love and devotion to the Supreme Personality of Godhead.

Krishna said very clearly that he will accept "a leaf, a flower, fruit or water." He specifically does not include meat, fish or eggs in the list; therefore a devotee does not offer them to Him. Out of love, the devotee offers Krishna only the purest and choicest foods and these certainly do not include the weeks-old-rotting corpses of slaughtered animals or the potential embryos of chickens. In most religious systems people ask God to feed them, but in Krishna Consciousness the devotee offers food to God as an expression of love for Him. Even in ordinary dealings, somebody will prepare a meal as a sign of love and affection. It isn't only the meal itself that is appreciated, but the pure love and consideration that goes into it. In the same way, the process of offering food to God is intended to help us increase our affection and devotion toward Him.

KASTURI SANDESH
PISTACHIO CHEESE FUDGE WITH ROSE WATER

This is one of Krishna's favorite sweets and is typical of those offered to Him in the temples around India every day.

Known also as "Royal Sandesh," this sweetmeat is flavored and colored with four distinctive ingredients: crushed cardamom seeds, saffron threads, minced pistachios and rose water. The cardamom and saffron are kneaded into the cheese along with the sugar and, sitting for 24 hours, the flavors intensify. The pistachios provide a pale green blanket of color. Before serving, the cake is sprinkled with rose water, then cut into squares. Each square is garnished with a small piece of a brilliant pink or red rose petal. Preparation and cooking time (after the chenna is made, drained and pressed for 15 minutes): 45 minutes. Makes: about 1 pound (455 g)

freshly made chenna cheese (pag 315) made from 10 cups (2.5 liters) whole milk
1/2 cup (110g) superfine sugar
1/2 tbs. (7 ml) cardamom seeds, coarsely crushed
a pinch of good-quality saffron threads

1/4 cup (35 g) blanched raw pistachios, minced
1/2 tbs (7 ml) rose water
a few insecticide-free garden pink or red rose petals (optional)

Unwrap the warm pressed chenna and transfer to a clean countertop, thoroughly blend in the sugar, cardamom seeds and saffron, and bray the cheese until it is without a touch of graininess.

Place a heavy-bottomed pan over the lowest possible heat, add the cheese until it is without a touch of graininess.

Place a heavy-bottomed pan over the lowest possible heat, add the cheese, and stirring constantly with a wooden spoon, cook for 10-15 minutes or until the surface becomes slightly glossy and the texture is slightly thickened. (The cheese will continue to turn up as it cools.)

Scrape the sandesh onto a buttered tray and press it into a flat 1 inch (2.5) thick cake pan. Set it aside to cool. While still warm, sprinkle with nuts and secure them in place by gently rolling the top with a rolling pin. When cool, cut the cake into 1-inch (2.5 cm) squares. When completely cool, store in single layers, separated with parchment or waxed paper in an airtight container. Refrigerated, they may be kept for up to four days.

> —from *Lord Krishna's Cuisine, The Art of Indian Vegetarian Cooking* by Yamuna Devi, E.P. Dutton-Bala Books 1987

=====

Rowena Pattee Kryder

Rowena is the author of seven published books, among them *Sacred Ground to Sacred Space, Emerald River of Compassion, Gaia Matrix Oracle* and *Destiny*. A former professor at the California Institute of Integral Studies in San Francisco, she has made five films and six videotapes and has exhibited her art widely in Europe and the U.S. She is also the founder, and now the program director, of the Creative Harmonics Institute, PO Box 940, Mount Shasta, California 96067, (916) 938-2484, fax: 938-2484.

"CHI offers year-round retreats and summer (week-long or more) intensives on 42 acres of pristine wilderness at the foot of Mount Shasta. The programs include meditation, art, shamanic work, sacred space, creativity, permaculture, as well as work with myth symbols and archetypes. Our main focus is creativity, which includes the steps of integrating tradition and vision, followed by manifestation and then release, which brings receptivity to new inspiration. Vegetarian meals are foundational in our way of life. 90% of the vegetables come directly from our vegetarian garden, and salads made with spinach, lettuce, kale, chard, carrots, beets, onions, parsley, and garlic are served at every meal. The following recipe is offered by our cook, Joyce Cochran."

> —R. P. Kryder

SOUTHERN STYLE SPICY KALE WITH VEGAN CORN BREAD

2 large onions
several cloves of garlic
3 tbs of olive oil
3 bunches of kale or mixed greens

6 tbs balsamic vinegar
1 tsp of crushed red pepper
1/5 tsp of seasalt and ground black pepper

Sauté onions in oil in a large skillet or wok. Add garlic, then greens. Toss them in the oil. Then add vinegar and seasonings; cover and cook briefly until wilted, then toss and cook until just tender.

VEGAN CORNBREAD

5 cups of cornmeal
1 cup of whole-wheat pastry
 flour
1 tsp of baking soda
2 tsp of baking powder

1/3 cup of honey
1/3 cup of canola oil
1 tsp of apple cider vinegar
3-4 cups of soy or rice milk.

Pre-heat oven to 420 degrees. Oil a large 10"x15" pan or large cast iron skillet, preheat pans in oven. In large bowl, stir the dry ingredients together. Then mix liquids together and add to dry ingredients. You may add grated carrots or zucchini. Turn into the pan and bake for 30 to 35 minutes.

---

k.d. lang, singer

"I grew up in cattle country—that's why I became a vegetarian. Meat stinks, for the animals, the environment, and your health."

CHILI CON TOFU

Chili:
1 pound crumbled tofu
1/2 tsp. garlic powder
1/2 tsp. chili powder
1 1/2 tsp. salt
2 tbs. oil
1 small diced onion
1 clove minced garlic
2 1/2 cups cooked pinto beans
4 tomatoes, skinned and
 chopped
1 small red or green pepper,
 deseeded and diced

1 can 8 oz corn or 8 oz baby
 corn

Sauce:
2 cups tomato sauce
1 cup pinto bean broth or
 water
2 tsps salt
1 tbs. tomato puree
pinch black pepper
1 tbs. chili powder
1 tsp. cumin

Stir together tofu, garlic powder, chili powder and salt. Heat onion and garlic in oil with tomatoes and peppers. Add tofu mixture and sauté until browned. Set aside. In saucepan, bring tomato sauce, bean broth, salt, pepper, chili powder and cumin to boil. Stir in tofu mixture, corn and beans and simmer until thoroughly heated.

Frances More Lappé

"She is the author of the epoch-making book, *Diet For a Small Planet.* Lappé admits that it was her sudden perception of the earth as a small and fragile planet that set her on the vegetarian path. Why food? In part she was influenced by the emerging ecology movement and the limits to growth consciousness. The first Earth Day was in 1970. The title as well as the tenor of Lappé's book captured the public's imagination as no previous vegetarian tract ever had. Its first edition sold over two million copies and its second edition, which was published in 1982, may far surpass it. As much as it is a serious discussion of ecology, geopolitics, economy and nutrition, the book also serves as a practical cookbook that the reader can use to reform his own eating habits and strike a blow for ecological sanity. It is ironic, yet appropriate, that the most successful debunker of what Lappé calls the Great American Steak Religion should have been born and bred in Texas, which is the capital of beef production in America."
—from *Famous Vegetarians* by Rynn Berry

SWEET AND PUNGENT VEGETABLE CURRY

2/3 cup soybeans, kidney
  beans, or limas (or a mix of
  the three)
1 cup brown rice
3/4 cup bulgur
2 or 3 tbs. oil for sauté
4 carrots, sliced diagonally
2 onions, thinly sliced
1 zucchini, sliced (optional)

1 tbs. hot curry powder (or
  more to taste)
1/4 cup flour
3/4 cup raisins
3/4 cup raw or roasted
  cashews
3 tbs. mango chutney (or
  more to taste)

Cook the beans and reserve one cup of the cooking liquid. Cook the brown rice and the bulgur. Heat oil and sauté carrots, onion, and zucchini until onions are translucent. Add curry powder and flour and sauté one minute. Add beans and reserved bean cooking liquid (or water) and simmer until carrots are tender but not soft. Add raisins, cashews, and chutney and more liquid if necessary (sauce should be thick). Taste for seasoning and simmer until raisins are soft. Serve over the cooked grain. Serves 6.

Joy Irene Lasseter, Ph. D.
Nutritional Consultant and Health Educator, author of vegetarian books. 3871 Piedmont Ave., Suite 360, Oakland   CA 94611

BAKED CINNAMON APPLE DELIGHT

**6 cups Rome red apples, sliced   overnight and drained
1 cup raisins, plumped (soak   1 tsp cinnamon
    in water, then drain)   1/2 teaspoon nutmeg, fresh
1 cup almonds, soaked   grated**

Fold ingredients together and pour into casserole dish. Add 2 tablespoons water into casserole and cover with lid. Bake at 350 until done (approximately 20 to 30 minutes). Serve in an elegant dessert dish. You can top with a dollop of yogurt.

Laura Lee
She hosts, from Seattle, The Laura Lee Show, a nationally syndicated Saturday night radio talk "For the Intellectually Daring". Call 1-800- 243-1438 for station near you.

SALAD LAURA LEE

Roast the vegetables.
Turn oven on to 400 degrees. In a large glass baking dish, chop into bite-size pieces one head cauliflower and one large onion. Spread

vegetables out to cover dish. If you are a garlic lover, lay on top one pod of garlic in the skin, with the top cut off. Add, if on hand, a couple of raw red or green chili peppers. Add 1/2 cup water to dish. Sprinkle French herbs liberally on top. Bake until vegetables become a bit browned, aromatic and tender, about 40 minutes. Remove from oven and let cool.

Prepare the Greens.
Into a very large salad bowl, chop one head of red leaf and one head of romaine (or your choice of lettuces). Add the roasted onion and cauliflower. Remove garlic from skin, dice, add. Dice roasted pepper with seeds and stem removed.

Dressing. Splash in the following:

1 tbs gomasio (Japanese seasoning of crushed sesame seeds and salt)	1 tsp raspberry vinegar 1 tbs tres classique red raspberry marinade
1 tsp tamari	1 dash dulse
1 tsp dried cilantro	

Toss. Serves 4.

━━━━━━━━━━━━

Leonardo Da Vinci
This is a translation made by Rynn Berry from the original Latin of a recipe in the cookbook from which Leonardo used to prepare his vegetarians meals—*De Honesta Voluptate*. It was written by Bartolomeo Platina in 1475 and is considered to be the first modern cookbook.

"Truly man is the king of beasts, for his brutality exceeds theirs. We live by the death of others. We are burial places!"

"I have from early age abjured the use of meat. The time will come when men such as I will look upon the murder of animals as they now look upon the murder of men."
—Leonardo da Vinci (1452-1519)

FRIED FIGS AND BEANS (FABA IN FIXORIO)

1 cup kidneys beans (soaked overnight and cooked)	garlic
1 cup sun-dried figs (chopped)	Kitchen herbs (basil, thyme, rosemary), salt and pepper
1 medium onion, chopped	to taste
sage	2 tbs. parsley, chopped fine.

In a greased frying pan combine cooked beans with onions, figs, sage, garlic, and various kitchen herbs. Fry well in oil. Sprinkle with aromatic herbs and serve. Serves four.

Mahavira

"No survey of vegetarians in history would be complete without paying homage to Mahavira, the historical founder of Jainism. Literally translated, the title or honorific Mahavira means the Great Man, or The Hero. After he attained complete knowledge (*kevala jnana*) at the age of 42, he was called *jina,* the conqueror (whence the name *Jain* is derived), which refers to the conquest of the self and soul purification achieved through his devotion to asceticism and *ahimsa* (non-injury to any living creature)."

—from *Famous Vegetarians* by Rynn Berry

Nobel Peace Prize winner Dr. Albert Schweitzer was a great admirer of Jainism. In fact, he was inspired by the Jain concept of *ahimsa* to coin his deathless phrase, "reverence for life."

SPICED GREEN BEANS (FALI)

1 1/2 lb. green beans	1/3 tsp turmeric powder
6 tbs oil	1/2 tsp garam masala
1 tsp cumin seeds	1 tsp salt (or to taste)
4 tsp coriander powder	

Wash and pick over the beans. Nip off the ends and cut the beans into one-half inch pieces. Heat the oil in a [heavy base] pot. Add the cumin seeds. When the cumin seeds start to sputter, add the beans and the remaining spices. Toss the beans and spices either with a spoon or by shaking the pot. Cover the pot and cook over a low flame. When the beans turn bright green, cook for two more minutes with the lid half-covering the pot. Remove from the burner when the beans are as cooked as you like them. Serves 4.

━━━━━━━━━━━

Paul & Linda McCartney

Linda: "We stopped eating meat many years ago. During the course of a Sunday lunch, we happened to look out of the kitchen window at our lambs playing happily in the fields. Glancing down at our plates, we suddenly realized that we were eating the leg of an animal who had until recently been playing in a field. We looked at each other and said, 'Wait a minute, we love these sheep—they are such gentle creatures. So why are we eating them?' It was the last time we ever did."

Paul: " What happens is that you realize that you really get into vegetarianism and start becoming an activist because you realize that what you're doing is helping to save these poor animals from getting shunted into a slaughterhouse."

SAVORY MINCE

1 lb butter or soy margarine	cups soya granules or 1 tin
1 large onion, chopped	nut mix
2 large potatoes, diced	Maggie seasoning or Marmite
1 packet soya mince or 1 1/2	2 vegetables soup stock cubes

Sauté onions, potatoes, and soya mince until light brown. Add enough water to cover. Bring to a boil and reduce heat. Then add the soup stock and the Maggie seasoning (or Marmite). Keep simmering until potatoes, onions, and soya mince are soft, and the water has been absorbed (approximately one-half hour). Serve with rice, or mashed potatoes, etc. Serves 4.

==========

Keith McHenry, Vegetarian Leader

He co-founded the international human rights group, Food Not Bombs, in 1980. The group can now be found in over 100 communities in North America, Europe and Australia, sharing free vegetarian food with the hungry. He was arrested 100 times in San Francisco and faced life in prison for supporting the rights of the poor. McHenry is an author, artist and outspoken critic of trans-national corporate greed and the new global austerity program. An American hero of food distribution, Keith has spent over 17 years promoting the vegetarian life style as a way to end hunger and disease.

TOFU CHEESE CAKE

3 1/2 cups tofu
1/4 cup water
1/2 cup melted margarine
1 1/2 fresh lemons juiced

3/4 cup honey, or maple sugar,
  if vegan
2 tsp vanilla

Crush tofu blocks in blender and add water. Mix in the other ingredients prior to blending. Mix into a very smooth, thick cream. Pour into granola crust. Bake for 30 minutes at 350° F.

Sprinkle with cinnamon, cool and refrigerate. Makes three 8-inch pies.

==========

Hayley Mills, actress

PASTA WITH FRESH TOMATOES

2 ripe large tomatoes cut into
  cubes
1 lb. brie cheese, cut into
  pieces (rind off)

3 garlic cloves minced
1 cup and 1 tbs. olive oil
1 cup cleaned fresh basil
  leaves cut into strips

2 1/2 tsp. pepper	and green pasta) fresh
1 1/2 lb. linguini (mix regular	grated parmesan cheese

Combine everything (except pasta, 1 tbs. oil and parmesan cheese) at least 2 1/2 hr. ahead of time (can even be combined in morning).

At mealtime cook linguini in water with 1 tbs. oil. Drain pasta when done. Mix well with the tomato/brie elixir, brie should melt.

Sprinkle with fresh parmesan. Serve warm. Enough for 4 people.

━━━━━━━━━━━━━━

Maria Rosaria Oaggio

She is an actress working in Italy for TV, cinema and theater. She's also been writing for radio and TV programs and has published several books.

MACCHERONI AND ZUCCHINI TRICOLORE

500 grams macaroni	5 spoonfuls of olive oil extra
1 small onion, finely chopped	virgin
50 grams parmesan cheese,	1 pinch grounded nutmeg
grated	7 leaves fresh basil
50 grams smoked cheese	1 small red tomato, not too
(caciocavallo, scamorza)	ripe
grated	salt and pepper to taste
100 grams ricotta or cottage	and lots of love and smiles (we
cheese	eat those as well)

In a large casserole heat up the oil and add the onion and sliced zucchini. Cook covered on a low flame for 15 minutes, then remove the lid and raise the flame to evaporate the excess water from the zucchini.

Cook the macaroni in a large amount of salted water for no more than 12 minutes. In the meantime, finely grate the parmesan and the smoked cheese. Drain the pasta and add it to the zucchini in their pot. Then add the grated cheeses and the ricotta, mixing gently with a wooden spoon.

Sprinkle with noce moscata and black pepper, then transfer the pasta to the serving plate and garnish with fresh basil leaves and slices of red tomato. Serves 4.

Buon appetito from Italy!

Brother Ron Picarski
Picarski is a Catholic Monk and a famous vegetarian chef.

MONASTIC SALAD

"This salad is truly monastic—simple, pure and wonderful..."
—Brother Ron

Serves 2 (as main course salad)

3 medium tomatoes, thinly sliced	**Dressing**
	6 tbs. extra virgin oil
1/2 pound fresh mushrooms, halved	6 Tbs. apple cider vinegar
	6 Tbs. water
1 1/2 cups sauerkraut	9 cloves minced garlic
1/2 cup diagonally sliced scallions	1 1/2 tbs. chopped parsley
	1 1/2 tsp. basil
green lettuce leaves and black olives for garnish	1 1/2 tsp. oregano
	1 1/2 tsp. sea salt
	1 tsp. Sucanat
	1/4 tsp. black pepper

In a large mixing bowl, combine the dressing ingredients and mix well. Add the tomato slices and mushrooms. Rinse the sauerkraut, lightly squeeze dry and add with the scallions to the dressing. Cover bowl and refrigerate overnight to marinate the vegetables and develop the flavors.

Serve cold on leaves of green lettuce and garnish with black olives.

This recipe has been excerpted from *Food for the Gods: Vegetarianism and The World's Religions* by Rynn Berry, Pythagorean Publishers, PO Box 8174, JAF Stn., New York, NY 10016.

Plato (427-347 B.C.)

He was one of the greatest ancient Greek philosophers and considered the founder of the European philosophical tradition.

HUMUS

1 cup chickpeas (soaked
  overnight and cooked)
2 tbs. finely chopped garlic
2 tbs. chopped parsley
juice of one lemon
1/2 cup tahini mixed with 1/3
  cup water

2 tbs. chopped dill
2 scallions, chopped
1 tbs. toasted sesame seeds
salt and pepper to taste
12 lettuce leaves

Let the chickpeas soak overnight. Then put them in a large skillet. Cover with water one-third of an inch above the chickpeas. Bring water to boil; then lower the flame and let simmer for one-and-a-half to two hours. Drain the peas and mash them with a fork. Add the remaining ingredients, except the lettuce, and mix them together thoroughly. Line the edge of each lettuce leaf with the humus, and roll it into a scroll.

Pythagoras (582-507 B.C.)

All students remember him for his "Theorem" but he is also considered in Western culture the father of vegetarianism. His philosophy reflects the influence of the Jains, the Indian brahmins and Egyptian teachers. Pythagoras taught that, through the transmigration of souls, all forms of animal life are interrelated. Precisely because the body of an animal may house the soul of a dear-departed relative, to eat its flesh would be considered an act of cruel cannibalism.

SAUTÉED CABBAGE WITH MUSTARD SEED

1 medium head cabbage cored	1 tsp. mustard seed
3 tbs. olive oil	salt and pepper to taste

Finely chop the cabbage. In a large skillet heat the olive oil and add the mustard seed, salt and pepper. As soon as the mustard seed starts to sputter, add the chopped cabbage. Cook over a high flame for five minutes, while stirring briskly to prevent scorching. Serve with whole grain bread. Serves 4.

In his *Natural History*, Pliny wrote that mustard, like cabbage, was highly esteemed by Pythagoras.

──────────

Lewis Regenstein

Lewis G. Regenstein is the president of The Interfaith Council for the Protection of Animals and Nature in Atlanta, Georgia, an affiliate of The Humane Society of the United States. He is the author of numerous newspaper and magazine articles on wildlife and the environment, and of such books as *Replenish the Earth: The Teachings of the World's Religions on Protecting Animals and Nature* (Crossroad, 1991); *Cleaning Up America the Poisoned: How to Survive our Polluted Society* (Acropolis, 1993); and *The Politics of Extinction: The Story of the World's Endangered Wildlife* (Macmillan, 1975).

WILD RICE WITH ROASTED PINE NUTS

2 cups wild rice, raw	1 large onion (vidalia in
3 tbs. olive oil	season)
2 tbs. corn oil margarine	1/4 cup cilantro
1 large garlic clove	1/2 cream cherry
1 can (approx. 14 1/2 oz)	salt pepper and paprika to
hearts of artichokes	your taste
2 large portobello mushrooms	
1 heaping cup pine nuts	

Steam rice in rice steamer for about 45 minutes. While rice is cooking, spray an iron skillet with non-stick spray and add margarine and two tablespoons of olive oil. Heat, then drop in onion, chopped very fine, and garlic, also chopped fine. Cook until light amber in color. Add hearts of artichokes, sliced 1/2 inch which have been cut into 8 pieces. Cook each for 2 minutes, then turn over mushroom and cook another 2 minutes. Remove from heat.

Add sherry, then stir entire contents into rice. Taste and leave over hot water until ready to serve. Serves 8.

John Robbins
Author of the best-sellers *Diet for a New America* and *May All Be Fed*. Founder, EarthSave International.

"A reduction in meat consumption is the most potent single act you can take to halt the destruction of our environment and preserve our precious natural resources."

QUICK & SIMPLE BANANA BREAD

Dry Ingredients:
2 cups whole wheat pastry
 flour
2 tbs. roasted grain beverage
 powder
1 tsp. baking soda
1 tsp. non-aluminum baking
 powder
1/2 tsp. fine sea salt

Moist Ingredients:
2 1/4 cup blended ripe
 bananas (about 5 average-
 sized bananas)
1/4 cup soy, rice or almond
 beverage
3 ounces safflower or canola
 oil
3 ounces maple syrup (2
 ounces, if bananas are
 extremely ripe)
1 cup chopped walnuts

Preheat oven to 350 degrees. Lightly oil an 8x8 baking pan (or equivalent). Mix dry ingredients in a large bowl. Blend moist ingredients in blender and then stir into dry ingredients. Mix in walnuts. Pour into baking pan and bake 30-35 minutes. Banana bread is done when a toothpick comes out clean.

=====

Steven J. Rosen is a widely respected religious scholar and author of *Diet for Transcendence.*

Diet for Transcendence presents its arguments in short, concise chapters that deal with each of the world's major religious traditions— Christianity, early Christianity, Judaism, Islam, Buddhism and Hinduism, touching briefly on the Zoroastrians, Sikhs and Jains. Rosen goes to the heart of the issue by searching the original scriptural texts of the world's various religious traditions. His important findings may be surprising. Not only do these traditions not require meat-eating but, quite to the contrary, extol the virtues of vegetarianism, considering it the highest standard of human diet.

VEGGIE CHOPPED LIVER

4 chopped medium size onions   1 tbs egg replacer
1 tsp turmeric   1/2 cup almonds
1 tsp canola oil   1/2 tsp of kelp
1/2 pound cooked mung beans

Sauté onions in oil; when ready, add all other ingredients and put in a food processor. Serve hot or cold. Serves 2.

=====

Ann Schaufuss

At 6 years of age, showing a natural ability for ballet, she was accepted into the Danish Royal Ballet. At seventeen she became Miss Denmark. Ann started modeling at twenty-two. Now, after more than 25 years, she represents a rare example of beauty and stability in a fashion world where thirty means old age. Her dynamic look has had an influence on other models who have chosen a vegetarian diet. "Almost 50% of the models I meet," Anne said, "are vegetarians, or they eat very little meat. I think it is a good direction."

In the early seventies, Ann was introduced to vegetarianism by former Beatle George Harrison, a close friend of Clive Arrowsmith, the photographer she was living with at the time. Harrison introduced both of them to yoga and Krishna Consciousness. Working as a fashion model and in commercials, she has been appearing regularly on TV programs and on the covers of Vogue, Officiel, Elle, Paris Match and many other magazines all over the world.

For many years Ann donated a good part of her income to charity programs. We wish her the longest career and thank her and other vegetarian models for never compromising, always rejecting advertisement work for meat, fur or products related to cruelty or suffering.

The mother of a healthy vegetarian child, vegetarian by birth, Ann looks much younger than her age. Now, she is starting a new career as a healer. After many years of studying and practice, Ann is teaching how to reach equilibrium and develop personal power through relaxation.

"Vegetarianism," said Ann, "has been my beauty secret and the following recipe is healthy and will keep you in a good shape."

Sunny Coconut Rice

tofu for 4 persons
2 cups of white basmati rice
3 cups of water
salt to taste

Coconut Gravy:
milk 400 grams
2 cans of coconut cream
little asafetida or 1 onion
2 tsp. curry powder
salt and pepper to taste

Boil the water and add salt, put in the washed rice, bring back to boil and turn down the heat. Cover with well-fitting lid and let stand 6-8 minutes until all the water has gone. In the meantime, heat your tofu. In a big frying pan, mix a little butter with some asafetida. If onion is used, it should be fried gently in the butter. Then pour in the 2 cans of coconut milk, stir in the curry powder and let simmer down to 3/4 of original volume. Salt and pepper to taste and serve over rice and tofu. Serves 4.

George Bernard Shaw

"Author of more than thirty plays that have become classics of the modern theater, Shaw also distinguished himself by turns as one of the greatest drama and music critics ever to have put pen on paper. In 1925, he was awarded the Nobel Prize for literature. Coincidentally, it was Shaw's vegetarianism that put him on the way to getting his first steady job as a writer. Through his friendship with Henry Salt—whose pamphlet, *A Plea for Vegetarianism*, had persuaded Gandhi not to renounce vegetarianism—Shaw was introduced to William Archer, the literary critic for *Pall Mall Gazette*. Archer began sending Shaw books to review. So witty, so penetrating, so stylishly written were Shaw's reviews that they quickly became the talk of London. Before long, rival papers were bidding for his services and, under his own name as well as a nom de plume, he began writing music and drama critiques for the *London Star* and the *Saturday Review* that are regarded as masterpieces of their genre."

—from *Famous Vegetarians* by Rynn Berry

CASSEROLE OF BRUSSELS SPROUTS

1 1/2 lb Brussels sprouts
1 medium onion
butter or soy margarine
5 medium tomatoes

1 cup cheddar cheese or 1 cup cheddar-style soy cheese (made from soybeans), grated (optional).

Prepare Brussels sprouts (pick over, wash, and trim). Preheat oven to 325 degrees. Slice onion and sauté in a little butter (or margarine) until transparent. Scald, peel, and slice tomatoes.

Arrange sprouts in casserole with onions and tomatoes. Add very little water—about one-half cup.

Cover and bake in an oven for forty-five minutes. When sprouts are tender, sprinkle with grated cheese or soy cheese, and place under broiler until golden brown. Serves four.

This recipe appears in *The George Bernard Shaw Vegetarian Cookbook* by Alice Laden and R. J. Minney, Taplinger Publishing Co. Inc. 1972.

Song of Peace

"We are the living graves of murdered beasts,
Slaughtered to satisfy our appetites,
We never pause to wonder at our feasts,
If animals, like men, can possibly have rights.
We pray on Sundays that we may have light
To guide our footsteps on the path we tread;
We are sick of war, we don't want to fight,
The thought of it now fills our hearts with dread,
And yet we gorge ourselves upon the dead.
Like carrion crows, we live and feed on meat,
Regardless of the suffering and pain
We cause by doing so. If thus we treat
Defenseless animals for sport or gain,
How can we hope in this world to attain
The PEACE we say we are so anxious for?
We pray for it, o'er hecatombs of slain,
To God, while outraging the moral law,
Thus cruelty begets its offspring—WAR."
—George Bernard Shaw (1865-1950)

William Roy Shurtleff

Database producer, publisher, author, librarian, archivist and director of Soyfoods Center, P.O. Box 234 (1021 Dolores Dr.), Lafayette, California 94549-0234 USA. Phone:(510) 283-2991. Fax:(510) 283-9091

The "Soyfoods Center" is the world's leading source of information on soyfoods. Shurtleff, a vegetarian genius, has put together the VegeScan, the world's most comprehensive computerized bibliographic database relating to all aspects of vegetarianism and veganism worldwide, from 238 B.C. to the present. Unsurpassed for doing a review of the literature in any field relating to vegetarianism (history of vegetarianism, health and medical aspects, cookbooks, nutritional information, philosophical and ethical aspects, planning the diet, athletics and endurance, infants and children, institutional food service), the VegeScan database has a strong historical orientation, plus a wealth of the most current references from around the world, updated daily.

WONDERFUL CREAMY TOFU DIP OR DRESSING:
OUR FAVORITE LATEST DISCOVERY

10 ounces tofu	**2 tbs minced pickles**
1/4 or 1/2 cup oil	**1 tbs minced onion**
2 tbs lemon juice	**1/2 tbs prepared mustard**
1 1/2 tbs honey	**1/2 tsp salt**
1/4 cup minced parsley	

Combine all ingredients in a blender and puree for 30 to 60 seconds, or until smooth. Great with chips, or sticks of freshly sliced carrots, green peppers, jicama, cucumbers, cauliflower, cherry tomatoes, Jerusalem artichoke, or celery. Note: the amount of oil may be reduced to taste. Makes 2 cups

Soyfoods
Protein source of the future...now.

Like a growing number of scientists, experts on world food supplies, agricultural economists and nutritionists, we feel that soybeans will be one of the key protein sources for the future on Planet Earth. One of the world's great renewable resources, soy holds great promise to meet great needs. Here are ten good reasons why:

1) **Lowest Cost:** Soybeans are presently the least expensive source of protein in virtually every country around the world.

2) **Optimum Land Utilization:** A given area of land planted with soybeans can produce much more usable protein than if planted with any other conventional farm crop and twenty times as much as if the land were used to raise beef cattle or grow their fodder.

3) **High Nutritional Value:** Soyfoods are a rich source of high-quality complete protein, with a protein quality equal to that found in

chicken or beef. They are low in calories and saturated fats, and completely free of cholesterol.

4) **Time Tested:** For over two thousand years, soyfoods have served as a key protein source for more than one-fourth of the world's population.

5) **Remarkably Versatile:** The soybean yields a cornucopia of delicious foods, including tofu (the world's most popular soyfood), tempeh, soymilk, miso, shoyu or soy sauce, soy flour, soy nuts, fresh green soybeans, textured soy protein (TVP), and various meat analogues.

6) **Appropriate Technology:** Most of these foods can be produced in cottage industries, using appropriate technology, as well as in modern factories.

7) **New Dairylike Products:** Soybeans yield an array of high-quality, low-cost, healthful dairylike products: Soymilk, yogurt, ice cream, cheese, etc.

8) **Hardy and Adaptive:** Soybeans can be grown under a wide range of climatic conditions and are quite resistant to pests, diseases and drought.

9) **Free Nitrogen Fertilizer:** A legume, the soybean enriches the soil with free nitrogen fertilizer—a key fact, since the price of chemical fertilizers has quadrupled since 1973.

10) **Great Productivity Potential:** Worldwide production of soybeans continues to skyrocket, having more than doubled in the past decade. Soybeans could now provide 25 percent of the yearly protein needs of every person in the world.

Thus, soyfoods can serve as an ideal protein backbone for the diet of health-minded, cost-conscious people who love fine foods.

Isaac Bashevis Singer

"Born in 1904, in Radzymin, Poland, Singer had wanted to become a vegetarian as a child, but his father, who was an orthodox rabbi, would have none of it. He scolded Singer for wanting to be holier than Yaweh, who, with his appetite for animal sacrifices in the Old Testament, was obviously no vegetarian. Chastened, Singer put off his conversion to a more propitious time—some fifty years later. At twenty-one he rewrote the Ten Commandments so as to include the eleventh—'Do not kill nor exploit the animal, don't eat its flesh, don't flail its hide, don't force it to do things against its nature.'

"His earliest novel, written in 1935, *Satan in Goray*, contains vegetarian leitmotifs, as do many of his other novels and stories. When asked about this, Singer said that the vegetarian themes came out of his pen automatically, and that the eating of meat has always bothered him. After George Bernard Shaw, he is the second Nobel Prize winning author in history to be a vegetarian."

—from *Famous Vegetarians* by Rynn Berry

When people used to ask him if he was vegetarian for health reasons, Singer answered promptly: I want the chicken to be healthy.

KASHA WITH ONIONS

3 tbs vegetable oil
3 onions chopped
1 cup buckwheat groats
2 cups boiling water

1 tsp sea salt or Vegesal
1 large dollop butter or soya
   margarine per serving

Fry onion in oil until golden. Add buckwheat groats and sauté until the onions turn darker. Pour on the boiling water, and let simmer over low flame for about fifteen minutes. Serve with a large dollop of butter or soya margarine. Serves 4-6.

───────────────

Seth Spellman III is a vegetarian lawyer, 8028 Inverness Ridge Rd., Potomac MD 20854.

"A lot of people are surprised when a jury returns a verdict which seems so contradictory to the evidence presented in a case. Not I. Nothing surprises me anymore. Am I just jaded by years of practice in a less than perfect legal system? No, my feelings are based on common sense observation of people in general. Take meat eating for example. The case against meat eating is rock solid. It's inconsistent with human physiology, an ecological disaster, economically impractical, and inconceivably cruel. Yet, consumption of meat is growing. Does anyone ever stop to consider the evidence? Perhaps when people clear their consciousness with respect to the clear case against meat eating, they can be expected to render better judgment in the courtroom."

—Seth Spellman

CHIDWA
Preparation time: 1 1/4 hours. Serves 10

1 tablespoon fennel seeds	1/4/ cup raisins
1/2 teaspoon turmeric	1 1/4 cups flat rice
1/2 teaspoon cayenne pepper	1/2 cup cashews
1 1/4 teaspoons salt	1 large baking potato, peeled,
1 1/2 tablespoons sugar	coarsely shredded
1 tablespoon ajwain	soak in cold water 1/2 hour,
2 hot green chilies, seeded and	drain and pat dry
minced	vegetable oil for deep frying

In a small frying pan roast the fennel seed over a medium flame until they turn a few shades darker. Remove from flame and set aside.

In a small bowl combine the turmeric, cayenne pepper, salt, sugar, ajwain, and chilies and set aside.

Line two plates with several paper towels and keep them near the frying area

Heat the vegetable oil in a wok or saucepan over a high flame. Drop in a handful of shredded potato, stirring occasionally until it is a golden brown. Remove with slotted spoon and drain on the paper towels. Fry the remainder of the potatoes the same way.

Reduce the flame to medium. Place a handful of flat rice in a metal strainer and lower it into the hot oil. Within a minute the frothing will settle. The flat rice is done when it is crisp but not brown. Remove the strainer and place the flat rice on the paper towels to drain. Fry the remaining flat rice in the same way.

Fry the cashews in the same manner as the flat rice until they are golden brown. After all the ingredients have cooled to room temperature, mix them together in a mixing bowl. Add the fennel seeds, raisins, and spice mixture and mix well. Store in an air-tight container.

Leo Tolstoy
Author, ascetic

SOUPE PRINTANIERE

1/4 cup carrots, diced	**(3 vegetable bouillon cubes**
1/4 cup turnips, diced	**dissolved in 1 1/2 quarts of**
1/2 cup green beans, cut into	**water)**
half inch lengths	**parsley, or chervil for**
1/2 cup fresh green peas	**seasoning**
1 1/2 quarts vegetable broth	**salt and pepper to taste.**

Prepare vegetables. Steam or boil each vegetable separately in one-half inch of water for ten minutes until tender. Drain and add to boiling vegetable broth. After it has resumed boiling, lower heat and simmer for a few minutes. Remove from flame and add seasonings. Serves 6.

Quotes from Tolstoy

The Highest Spiritual Capacity
"Man suppresses in himself the highest spiritual capacity—that of

sympathy and pity towards living creatures like himself—and by violating his own feelings becomes cruel."

The Living Graves
"While our bodies are the living graves of murdered animals, how can we expect any ideal conditions on earth?"

Special Joy
"The progress of the vegetarian movement should cause special joy to those whose life lies in the effort to bring about the Kingdom of God on earth, not because vegetarianism is in itself an important step towards that kingdom, but because it is a sign that the aspiration of mankind towards moral perfection is serious and sincere."

Claudio Vannini
Known as Rome's most prominent vegetarian guru, Claudio Vannini is now in charge of three vegetarian restaurants in the capital city of Italy (Rome).

1975 - The activities of the Italian Macrobiotic Center start in Rome.

1980 - Opening of the Margutta Vegetariano, the first vegetarian restaurant in Italy, that soon became most well-known and well-attended by politicians and celebrities: Federico Fellini, Giulietta Masina, Marcello Mastroianni, Isabella e Renzo Rossellini.

1988 - Opening of the Antico Bottaro, elegant version of the Margutta, where to have a candlelight dinner and meet international celebrities and stars like Michael Bolton and Claudio Baglioni.

1993 - Opening of the Supernatural, the first vegetarian pizzeria and "hamburgheria," in the center of Rome. With original dishes and high quality biologic products, it rapidly gained wide success, to the point of being now re-proposed in franchising. For more information about the franchise project, contact Claudio Vannini, c/o Supernatural.

Margutta Vegetariano - Via Margutta 118, 00187 Roma
Tel. 6/32650577
Antico Bottaro - Passeggiata di Ripetta 15, 00186 Roma
Tel. 6/32650577
Supernatural - Via del Leoncino 38, 00187 Roma Tel. 6/32650577

VEGETARIAN GOULASH

1 bottle wet seitan, cut in
   large chunks
1 1/2 kilos onions
2 medium size carrots
250 grams peeled tomatoes
1 clove garlic
1 celery
4 tbs balsamic vinegar
1/2 glass fresh cream
1 can beer (regular or non
   alcoholic)

vegetable broth (as needed)
4 tsp hot paprika
3 grams marjoram
3 grams thyme
5 bay leaves
1 small branch rosemary
salt to taste
extra virgin olive oil (as
   needed)

Peel the onions and blend till creamed. Mix in a pan with oil, garlic, bay leaves and rosemary. Fry for about 20 minutes, adding broth as much as required.

Add celery and carrots, not too finely chopped. Then pour in seitan in chunks with all its liquid, all the remaining spices and the peeled tomatoes, slightly mashed with a fork.

Allow to cook for about ten minutes, then add the other ingredients in the following order: beer, vinegar and, after a few minutes, the cream. Keep cooking for another 5 minutes, stirring all the time. Serves 4.

Linda Vephula
Publisher

"Angels—almost overnight, everywhere you look you see or hear about angels. The angel phenomenon is sweeping across the country and in fact around the world. There are retail stores stocked with angel merchandise, book stores lined with angel books, network angel television shows, angel documentaries, newspaper articles, radio shows…the list goes on! Why? Why now? Is it commercialism or is there a deeper true reason?"

To answer all these questions, Linda Whitmon Vephula started a wonderful magazine: *Angel Times*. She is not affiliated with any particular church, religious denomination or religion. She sees angels being expressed in all the religions of the world. They are messengers of love, overriding the differences in religious interpretation and a common denominator among the world's religions.

To find out more about *Angel Times*, call 800-865-5771 or 404 986-9787. *Angel Times*, Suite 400, 4360 Chamblee-Dunwoody Road, Atlanta GA 30341 USA.

HARK THE CHERRY ANGEL RING

1-17 oz can pitted bing cherries, drained with juice reserved

13 oz package Kosher cherry gelatin (kosher gelatin is not made from animal products like regular gelatin and it is found in the international section of many grocery stores)

1-12 oz carton frozen lowfat whipped topping, thawed

1 prepared angel food cake, torn in small pieces.

Candied or other cherry halves for decorating (optional).

In 2-cup glass measure, place cherry juice and add water to make 1 cup.

Heat to boiling and stir in gelatin until dissolved. Transfer to large bowl. Stir in cherries and chill until partially set. Fold in 2 cups whipped topping. Put one layer of torn cake in bottom of angel food pan. Cover with layer of cherry mixture, then repeat layers. With rubber spatula push cake so sauce covers all cake pieces.

Refrigerate 6 hours or more. Un-mold cake and frost with remaining whipped cream. Arrange cherries on top, if desired.

━━━━━━━━━━

Lailah Wah, R.Ac. (NCCA) is an expert on healing wisdom, acupuncture, herbology, moxabustion, Shiatsu, Bach Flower, homeopathy, and life style counseling. She is located in The Lewis Tower Building, 225 South 15th Street, Suite 1400, Philadelphia PA 19102 (215) 731-0177.

SPINACH FRITTATA DI COUNTLESS VENUTI

2 lb. spinach or 4 packages of
   frozen spinach
1 cup ricotta cheese
1/2 cup of romano or parmesan cheese, roughly grated
olive oil
1/4 cup Jarlsburg or cheddar
   cheese (sharp)

6-8 Italian green peppers
1/2 cup chopped Italian
   parsley
1/2 cup chopped basil
1/4 cup cilantro (optional)
1/4 cup pine nuts
1 cup cooked rice
2 medium sized tomatoes

Generously pour the olive oil into the pie dishes. Entirely cover the bottom of the pan. Slice Italian green peppers in half lengthwise and line the pie dishes. Place in the oven and cook at 350 degrees for 15 minutes or until par-cooked.

Steam the fresh spinach, then chop it coarsely. Add all ingredients except the tomatoes. Pour mixture over the par-cooked peppers and bake at 350 degrees. Before frittata becomes firm, remove from oven and place tomato slices on top of pie. Place back into oven. Cook until the edges become golden brown.

Spinach Frittata may be served hot or room temperature. Yields two 9" pies.

Dennis Weaver, actor

AVOCADO TOMATO SANDWICH

seven-grain coarse bread
soy margarine
strips of avocado
sliced tomato

sunflower seeds and/or
   sprouts
thin slice of mozzarella-style
   soy cheese

Spread two slices of coarse, whole grain bread with soy margarine. On one slice, make a layer of avocado strips. Next, add a layer of sunflower seeds and/or sprouts. Then add a layer of sliced tomato and cheese. Use a bit of mustard for added zest. Cover with other bread slice.

Paramahamsa Yogananda

Sri Durga Mata shared many experiences she had as an intensely close disciple of Paramahansa Yogananda. In her book, *A Paramahansa Yogananda Trilogy of Divine Love*, she mentions many of his favorite pastimes, one of which was cooking. One dish he often prepared was Saffron Rice. She never mentioned exact recipes in her writings of Yogananda, but would list basic ingredients. The following recipe comes from many attempts made by Kay Vontillius at getting it just right. We believe Yogananda would be pleased.

GURUJI'S SAFFRON RICE

2 tbs ghee
1 cup white basmati rice
2/3 cup raw almonds
  (chopped in blender for 15
  seconds)
3 cinnamon sticks
2 bay leaves
2 cups water
dash sea salt

2/3 cup golden raisins
1/4 gram Spanish saffron
  strings
1/3 cup sugar (just to taste)

Heat ghee to medium temperature in a stainless steel pot. Add basmati rice, cinnamon sticks, chopped almonds, and bay leaves. Sauté and stir until rice is shiny. Add water, sea salt, raisins and saffron. Stir until boiling. Reduce heat to a simmer. Cover and cook for 20 minutes. Add sugar, stir, cover and let sit until you are ready to serve to your most beloved. Suggested drink: fresh organic apple juice with a dash of nutmeg.

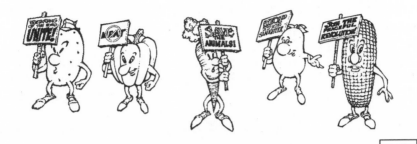

Recipes of
Vegetarian Groups

We Need Movements

"Without movements for social change, we would still have: legalized slavery, child labor, no voting rights for women, segregation, and involuntary human experiments. We can raise our collective voices to change the situation for animals, too. You can start by adopting this motto: Animals are not ours to eat, wear, experiment on or use for entertainment."
—from *PETA* magazine

The American Anti-Vivisection Society
801 Old York Road, Suite 204
Jenkintown, PA 19046-1685
(215) 887-0816, Fax (215) 887-2088

The AAVS is an international organization that affirms that the use of animals in research, testing and education is morally objectionable. Vivisection actually harms people, as well as animals, by wasting time, effort and money on research of little or no benefit. Non-animal scientific research, however, holds great promise for treating and curing both human and animal ailments.

"Every year millions of animals are killed in experiments to supposedly safety-test the products we use. While these tests are not required by law, and there are many viable alternatives, the practice still continues. Animals used in product testing are force-fed hazardous substances such as weed killers, insecticides, drugs and oven cleaners. They have lipstick and hair dye poured in their eyes. They have caustic cleaning products burn holes through their skin. They are forced to inhale cigarette smoke and chemical fumes. They are shot and used for germ warfare experiments by the military. The ways animals are used in product testing are endless. All of these experiments are unnecessary and the results can often be misleading. The findings from these tests rarely tell us anything of actual benefit to human beings. Non-human animals respond very differently than humans do to most substances and procedures, which makes the extrapolation of results from one species to another very difficult. Many products have been withdrawn from the market because of dangerous side effects, which were not revealed despite extensive tests on animals. We are led to believe that without animal experiments we cannot survive. The facts show otherwise."

—from the *AV* magazine

SIKORA'S SCRUMPTIOUS CORN BREAD

1 cup cornmeal	1 tsp. baking soda
1 cup whole wheat flour	1/2 cup maple syrup
1 cup soy milk	1/2 cup margarine
1/2 tsp. salt	

Mix all ingredients. Pour into greased 8x8 pan. Drizzle with molasses. Bake 25 minutes at 425 degrees. This is the yummiest corn bread you will ever eat.

The American Vegan Society
P.O. Box H
Malaga, NJ 08328-0908
56 Dinshah Lane (from West Blvd., S. on Dinshah Drive)
phone: (609) 694-2887

The American Vegan Society, founded 1960, advocates a diet without any animal product (no meat, fish, fowl; no animal broth, fat or gelatin; no eggs, milk, or cheese; no honey) on ethical and healthful grounds, and a life style excluding use of animal products such as fur, leather, wool, or silk—notably in items of clothing. Vegans also make efforts to avoid use of toiletries, cosmetics, household goods, and other commodities that contain often less-than-obvious animal ingredients, oils, secretions, hormones, etc. Vegans enjoy a varied and nutritious diet from the plant kingdom—a delightful range of tasty dishes and substitutes for commonly eaten items. The variety of acceptable clothing, etc. is increasing, attractive and serviceable. AVS publishes *Ahimsa* magazine, quarterly ($18 per year), featuring in-depth articles on all aspects of veganism. AVS has a mail order book, video and literature service with an extensive lists of books on veganism, vegetarianism, animal rights and health.

Alternatives to Dairy Products and Eggs
by Freya Dinshah

A growing number of people are coming to recognize their need to stop using eggs and dairy foods, prompted by what they learn about the life and death of farm animals, and because of health concerns.

Making such a decision is a major first step. The next step is an adjustment in eating habits, and finding ways to fill the gaps left at breakfast, lunch, dinner and snack times. Specific alternatives can be a big help.

Milk as a beverage, is replaced by drinks made from soy, rice, oats, almonds, etc., either from one of these items or from a combination. Simple, inexpensive drinks can be made at home (see vegan cookbooks). The range of commercially produced soy and/or rice beverages is making it easy for many people to stop drinking cow milk.

Check out your supermarket or health food store for the commercial products by companies such as Eden Foods (800/248-0320), Imagine Foods (415/327-1444), Pacific Foods (503/692-9666), and Westbrae (310/886-8200 ext 124).

Cheese lovers will fare best working in their kitchens with *The Uncheese Cookbook* by Joanne Stepaniak, which presents an array of vegan versions of familiar cheeses and cheese dishes. Key ingredients are nuts, seeds, and nutritional yeast (a food yeast with a cheesy taste) and starchy thickeners, sometimes beans or tofu. Examples of flavorings are mustard, onion, garlic and spices. Unfortunately, most of the "non-dairy" cheeses currently sold contain casein, a protein component of milk, which is responsible for the shredding and melting quality of cheese, and imparts these attributes to the majority of so-called "non-dairy" cheeses. Some contain other animal-derived ingredients also.

Galaxy (800/441-9419) distributes Soymage, without casein. A recent market entry from Sharon's Finest (707/576-7050) is VeganRella (one of their cheese-alternatives). The limited number of off-the-shelf, truly vegan cheese simulators can be supplemented by bean dips and spreads. Humus (made from chick peas or garbanzos, tahini, lemon juice, oil, flavorings and seasonings) is one example; but the range of possibilities increases greatly if you improvise and use other peas, beans or lentils. A simple and delicious alternative is provided by the avocado. Also there are many nut and seed butters from which to choose.

Eggs can be easily omitted from the diet. Scrambled tofu is just as quick and easy to prepare as scrambled eggs. Cooked yellow split peas (either "soft" or "firm") can be eaten occasionally. According to Joann Sisco, owner of Integrity Baking (609/694-4235) which markets an all-vegan line of cookies, cakes, etc., pancakes and cakes can be made easily without eggs. For those who feel the need for egg-substitutes when they cook, first consider what attribute you are seeking: binding can be accomplished using arrowroot starch, potato starch, or corn starch, oat flour or wheat flour, quick oats, mashed potato, or quick-cooking tapioca; lightness can be achieved by using some extra yeast or baking soda, and by using fruit juice or tomato juice to replace some or all of the liquid in a recipe. You can also use soft whole-wheat pastry flour in place of, or in addition to, whole-wheat flour for cakes.

In bread, a little vital gluten (about 1/4 cup for 8 cups flour) is the secret.

Ener-G Foods (800/331-5222) markets powdered Egg-Replacer. Other egg-replacer formulas are:

1) 1 tsp. arrowroot powder + 1 tsp. soy powder + 1/4 cup water.
2) 1/4 cup soaked soybeans or garbanzos blended with an equal amount of water.
3) 1 tbs. tahini + 3 Tbs. liquid.
4) 2 oz. tofu blended with liquid in recipe.
5) A half banana, mashed.
6) 4 tbs. of 1 part freshly ground flaxseed + 3 parts water (or liquid listed in recipe) stirred or blended together. As the mixture stands off for a while, it becomes thicker or stiffer.

Butter in cooking can be replaced by vegetable oil, etc.; there are all-vegetable soy margarines such as Shedd's Willow Run Spread (Van Den Bergh 800/735-3554), Hain Margarine (213/5848311). Fruit puree can replace some of the fat generally used in baking. Cooked grains blended smooth with a nut or seed butter are a good spread on bread and are better for health in terms of saturated fats, trans-fats, and cholesterol.

Mayonnaise replacements can be made with recipes utilizing tofu, or cooked potato, or nut-milk. Nasoya Foods (508-537-0713) markets a well-marketed Nayonnaise.

Ice Cream now has many rivals in the frozen dessert field. Some suitable for vegans are made by companies such as Imagine Food and Turtle Mountain (503-998-6778). Frozen bananas have a central role in many home-made "ice-creams".

Vegan puddings can also be found from Imagine Foods. There are soy yogurts too; one company making them is White Wave (303/443-3470). Or you can whip up a fresh and delightful smoothie in your blender, using fruit and tofu, and/or soy milk, and optional nuts.

Revised from *Ahimsa* magazine #36-03, published by AVS.

Recipes from *The Vegan Kitchen* by Freya Dinshah.

HOLIDAY YAMS

Filling:

2 lb. yams, cooked & peeled	7 oz wt chopped pitted dates
1-1/2 apples	1 tbs. oil
1 (14 oz) can unsweetened pineapple chunks	**Topping**
	3/4 cup rolled oats
Sauce:	3 tbs. oil
1-1/2 cups pineapple juice (from chunks, plus extra)	1/4 cup unsweetened, shredded coconut

Simmer ingredients for sauce, stirring often. Cook until dates are well softened and blend in. Slice yams and apple and mix with pineapple chunks. Gently stir in sauce. Place in large, oiled pie dish. Mix topping. Sprinkle over filling. Preheat oven to 400° F. Bake for 1 hour at 350° F. Serve hot or cold with ice cream.

ICE CREAM FAVORITE

Peel 3 large ripe bananas, removing any bruised spots. Cut in pieces and put in blender. Whizz it up. Nuts (2/3 cup raw cashew nuts) may be pre-ground in nut mill. Blend well on "high". Freeze 4-5 hours, or overnight. Serve with ice cream scoop.

Farm Animal Reform Movement
PO Box 30654, Bethesda, MD 20824

F.A.R.M. is a national, non-profit public interest organization, formed in 1981 by animal and consumer advocates to moderate and eliminate the destructive impacts of today's intensive animal agriculture on animal welfare, consumer health and environmental conservation. FARM seeks to achieve needed reforms through regulatory legislation and consumer boycott of animal foods. To this end, FARM conducts several national public education campaigns:

The Great American Meatout encourages Americans to kick the meat habit on March 20th to celebrate the coming of spring.

World Farm Animals Day is a worldwide observance held on Gandhi's birthday (October 2), memorializing the suffering and slaughter of billions of animals for food.

National Veal Ban Action seeks to ban the crate and anemic diet in raising veal calves.

CHOICE (Consumers for Healthy Option In Children's Education) is a nationwide effort to provide plant-based meals in public schools.

FARM operates from Washington through a national network of activists and support groups. It is funded by tax-deductible contributions from concerned individuals. Contributors receive periodic reports on national and local activities, and invitations to participate.

"...it is a sad fact that nutrition education in the U.S. is governed by commercial interests with sufficient clout to co-opt government agencies and the necessary funds to hire the public relations apparatus, rather than by a consensus of the nation's best nutritional minds. This situation cannot be allowed to continue and to degrade the health and welfare of the American people."
—Dr. Alex Hershaft

EGGPLANT MILANESE

1 quart tomato sauce	1 large onion, cut into rings
2 green peppers, sliced	3 large garlic cloves, diced
2 large eggplants, peeled and sliced	

Preheat oven to 350° F. In an 8"x12" baking pan, pour a thin layer of tomato sauce. Using 1 eggplant, add a layer of eggplant slices, one layer of all the onion rings, one layer of all the green peppers. Sprinkle diced garlic on top. Cover with tomato sauce, another layer of eggplant slices, and more sauce. Bake in the oven for approximately 1 hour, until vegetables are soft. Serves 4 to 6

Eating for Life

The reasons for adopting a plant-based diet vary. Most people do it out of concern for their health and longevity, but many are impressed by the cost savings, resource conservation, and reduced animal suffering. Getting started is easier than you may think. Plant-based food already makes up a large part of your diet, and meatless prepared foods are increasingly available. Take our menu suggestions, below, and the recipes inside, and combine them with your desire for a healthier, more compassionate diet. That's a recipe for LIFE!

Breakfast- Fresh fruit, Cereal with juice or soy milk, Breads or muffins, Apple sauce, Hot oatmeal with raisins, Pancakes or waffles

Lunch- Garden Salad (try adding fruits and nuts), Peanut butter, humus, or avocado sandwich, Vegetable soup with crackers, Topped baked potato, Pasta Salad, Bean burrito

Dinner- Spaghetti with tomato sauce, Grilled vegetables over rice Pasta tossed with vegetables, Veggie chili, Red beans and rice, Baked Eggplant

Dessert & Snacks- Fruit cobbler or pie, Nuts and raisins, Fruit salad, Carrot and celery sticks, Chips and salsa, Fresh fruit

---

Food Not Bombs

The message of this group is very simple and powerful: no one should be without food. The leaders of the planet—instead of spending every year trillions of dollars to produce and maintain weapons—should care for any hungry or malnourished person in need.

Food Not Bombs claims that the world produces enough food to feed everyone, if distributed equally. There is abundance of food. In the USA every day in every city, far more edible food is discarded than is needed to feed those who do not have enough to eat. Consider their point: before food reaches your table, it is produced and handled by farmers, co-ops, manufacturers, distributors, wholesalers and retailers. Some perfectly edible food is discarded for a variety of business reasons at every step. In the average city, approximately 10% of all solid waste is food. This is an incredible total of 46 billion pounds nationally per year, or just under 200 pounds per person per year. Estimates indicate that only 4 billion pounds of food per year would be required to completely end hunger in America, and there is clearly an abundance of edible, recoverable food being thrown away. For more information call 1-800-884-1136.

The Demographics of the Hungry

"Today, according to the Harvard School of Public Health, people living below the poverty line are going hungry at least once a month, and over 30 million people are going hungry on a regular basis. Astonishingly, less than 15% of the hungry are homeless. Moreover, the explosion of hunger has outstripped the ability of existing hunger relief programs, both governmental and private, to satisfy this crucial need.

Many do not realize that the demographics of "The Hungry" have changed dramatically. Over the last decade, they have become:

Younger: 12.9 million (40%) are children, the true victims of this tragedy.

Poorer: 12.9 million (40%) live below the poverty line. This gap is widening as the real income of the bottom four-fifths of the American population continues to decrease.

More likely to be employed: 60% of poor families include workers, and the number of working hungry rose 50% from 1978 to 1986.

More likely to be female: 50% of poor families are headed by women.

Less likely to overcome poverty.

Clearly, the majority of people going hungry today are not the stereotyped street person as the media would have you believe. Hungry people are children and single parents (mostly women), the working poor, the unemployed, the elderly, the chronically ill, and those on a fixed income (such as veterans and people with physical and mental challenges/differences/disabilities). All of these people find themselves in the clutches of oppressive poverty even while trying to improve their condition."

—from *Food Not Bombs, How to Feed the Hungry and Build Community* by C.T. Lawrence Butler & Keith McHenry, New Society Publishers, 4527 Springfield Avenue, Philadelphia PA 19143.

TOFU SANDWICH SPREAD

Makes: 100 sandwiches. Equipment: medium mixing bowl, very large mixing bowl. Prep time: 2 hours

3 cups miso
3 cups water
8 cups tahini
25 lb. crumbled tofu
25 lemons, juice of

Optional:
1/2 cup garlic powder
8 cups diced onion
8 cups diced celery

Food Relief International
3450 S. Ocean Blvd.
Palm Beach, Florida 33480 USA
31a Lanark Rd., London W9 England

Founded and directed by Rytasha. Born in New York City into a wealthy and aristocratic family, she became a top international model and appeared in movies and on TV. After studying spirituality in all the different religions, in 1985, she gave up everything to work among "the poorest of the poor" in Bangladesh, India and Nepal. She is directing FRI, organizing charity programs and teaching that "the suffering of man would not change, until the consciousness of man will change. There is enough in the world for everyone's need but not for everyone's greed."

GREEN BEANS AND FRIED HOME MADE CHEESE
IN A THICK CREAMY CASHEW CILANTRO SAUCE

2 liters of whole milk
lemon juice from 2 lemons
1/2 kilo of stringless green
   beans, cut and steamed
1/2 cup of cashew nuts
1 inch of peeled minced ginger
2 or 3 green chilies seeded and
   minced
1/2 cup of fresh cilantro

500 gm of fresh natural
   yogurt
1 tbs. of ghee
1 tsp. of cumin seeds
6-7 fresh curry leaves
1 1/2 tsp. of salt or to taste
freshly grated nutmeg
freshly chopped cilantro to
   garnish

Place the milk to boil, stirring from time to time; when it starts to boil, turn off the heat and gradually add the lemon juice until the cheese separates from the whey. When the whey is clear, you have added enough. Place a double layer of cheesecloth in a sieve and strain your fresh cheese, folding the cloth over it and covering with heavy weight. Place the cheese on a draining sideboard while it presses, so that the excess whey can drain into the sink. Meanwhile, powder the cashew nuts in a blender, add the ginger, chilies, fresh cilantro and yogurt. Blend until smooth, then mix the beans with this sauce in a mixing bowl. Take a large, non-stick frying pan and heat the ghee over a medium flame. When it is hot, add the pressed cheese (which you can cut into 1 inch cubes) until they are golden on all sides. Remove with a slotted spoon and set aside. Now add the cumin seeds, followed by the fresh curry leaves, followed by the beans in their sauce. Continue simmering, adding the salt and some nutmeg as well as the fried cheese, until the sauce thickens. Serve hot, decorating with some fresh chopped cilantro.

How on Earth!

Teenagers are the fastest-growing group of vegetarians, say trend watchers. Young people who have gone (or are considering going) vegetarian should check out the quarterly publication of HOE. Their unique newsletter is for and by youth who support compassionate, ecologically-sound living. It covers a variety of environmental, animal and global issues, while encouraging activism and empower-ment among youth who are concerned about animals and the Earth. HOE recognizes that a vegetarian diet is an essential component of compassionate, sustainable living, so vegetarian recipes, nutritional advice, and life style information are important features of this newsletter.

Teenagers and young adults, ages 13-24, from the U.S. and Canada (even overseas), submit articles, art work, poetry, personal essays, vegetarian recipes, photography, and advice covering every-thing from current issues, to activism and boycotts, to dealing with parents and peers who just don't understand. You can subscribe to the newsletter, submit materials and volunteer to help out in various ways. HOE totally depends on youth involvement and provides a voice for young people's creativity, passion and concern for all life. HOW ON EARTH! celebrates every person's potential to make a difference. Everybody can subscribe to the newsletter: 1 year (4 issues) for $18. 1 year at Canadian rate for $21, postal money order. 2 years at special rate of $30 (8 issues). Write to HOW ON EARTH, P.O. Box 339, Oxford, PA 19363-0339, phone:(717) 529-8638

VEGETABLE PANCAKES

2 cups chopped vegetables **(cabbage, scallions, carrots, celery, etc.)**	**1 Tbs. soy sauce** **1 tsp. ginger powder** **(optional)**
1 cup unbleached white flour	**1 Tbs. oil**
1 cup water	

Mix all ingredients (except the oil) in large bowl. Heat oil in frying pan over medium heat. Form six pancakes and fry in oil on both sides until brown. After frying pancakes, lay them on a paper towel for a few minutes to drain off excess oil. Serves 2

The International Jewish Vegetarian Society

This Society, started in 1964, is supported by many eminent rabbinical authorities who are attached to, and take an active part in, the Society's endeavors. They publish regularly *The Jewish Vegetarian*. There are chapters and representatives throughout Europe, USA, Canada, South Africa, Australia and Israel. International Headquarters: Bet Teva, 855 Finchley Road, London NW11 8LX tel. & fax 0181-455-0692

Why a Jewish Vegetarian Society?

1) Because the original food man is ordered to eat in Genesis 1:29 is vegetarian: "Behold I give you every herb bearing seed and the fruit of every seed bearing tree for you it shall be for food."

2) Because permission to kill and eat animals was only granted as a result of man's evil and was accompanied with a curse (Genesis 9:5).

3) Because flesh foods are now the product of extreme cruelty, and contravene Tzar baal Chaim. Ninety-eight percent of all meat and poultry, kosher and non-kosher, comes from factory farms, contrary to many provisions of the Torah.

4) Injections of dangerous growth and sex change hormones, castrations and non-observance of the Sabbath (4th Commandment) mean that the flesh cannot be kosher. It is held that the laws of kasruth are a pathway back to the vegetarian way of life.

5) The Sabbatical year is one of our vital commands. Seventy-five percent of the world's grain and pulse is fed to the thousands of millions of artificially-bred animals. The Sabbatical year of rest for the land cannot be implemented if this unnatural population has to be fed. Under a vegetarian economy, the Sabbatical year could be observed without problems.

6) Nowhere in the Tenach is there a promise of flesh foods of any kind as a reward for keeping the commandments. The promise is always the gift of produce of the vines, the gardens and the fields. Sacrifice, according to Maimonides, was a concession to barbarism and to be phased out in man's gradual return to the Eden state.

SWEET AND SOUR CABBAGE AND APPLE SOUP

3/4 cup tomato juice
2 vegetable stock (bouillon)
  cubes
6-8 cups water
1/2 white cabbage, finely
  chopped
2 large cooking (tart) apples,
  chopped

1 medium onion, grated
  (shredded)
sea salt and freshly ground
  black pepper
juice of 1 lemon
honey, to taste

Boil together the tomato juice, vegetable stock (bouillon) cubes and water. Add the cabbage, apple and onion to the boiling mixture, reduce the heat and simmer for 1-2 hours until the cabbage is tender. Season to taste with sea salt and freshly ground black pepper, add the lemon juice and a teaspoon or so of honey to taste for a sweet-sour flavor, then serve hot.

From the Dachau Diary:

"I refuse to eat animals because I cannot nourish myself by the suffering and by the death of other creatures. I refuse to do so, because I suffered so painfully myself that I can feel the pains of others by recalling my own sufferings...I feel happy nobody wants me; nobody kills me; why should I, or would I, kill other creatures or cause them to be wounded or killed for my own pleasure and convenience."

—Edgar Kupfer-Koberwitz, Nazi Concentration Camp, Dachau, Germany

ISCOWP

The International Society for Cow Protection is organized to offer natural alternatives to present agricultural practices that support and depend on industrialization. Alternative energies offered by the cow and ox, ox training, a sound ecological agrarian lifestyle, and a lacto-vegetarian diet based on cruelty-free lifetime cow protection are the practices that ISCOWP would like to make available to everyone. In February 1991, ISCOWP began its first farm sanctuary in Efland, North Carolina. To become a member, send your annual membership fee of $15 to ISCOWP, 1299 A, Moundville WV. 26041. A written proposal, detailing ISCOWP's water resource development project, is available.

"Remember the Ox is the backbone of the farm, not the soup bone."
—Balabhadra dasa

OATMEAL CHIP COOKIES

1/2 cup butter	1 tsp. baking powder
1/3 cup oil	1 tsp. baking soda
1 cup brown sugar	1 tsp. salt
1/3 cup milk	3 cups oatmeal
1 tsp. vanilla	1 cup carob chips
2 1/2 cups flour	

Cream butter and oil together, then cream in the sugars. Add milk and vanilla. Beat until smooth. Beat in flour, baking powder, soda and salt. Mix, add oats and raisins and blend well. Bake at 350 degrees for about 15 minutes or until the undersides start turning brown. Makes about 3 dozen.

We suggest two other groups concerned for the well-being of cows:

Adopt A Cow, RD 1, Box 839, Port Royal, PA 17082 (707) 527-2476

Adopt-a-Cow is located at Gita-Nagari Farm in Port Royal, Pennsylvania. On the 350 acres, AAC currently supports 117 cows and oxen. AAC seeks to provide a living example of cow protection as described in the Vedas, allowing the animal to live its complete life span and thus avoiding the slaughterhouse. People are invited to come and see how AAC operates the farm, compared to the standard dairy or beef farm. The adoption plans allow people to "adopt a cow" by giving a monthly donation of $30, which covers the cost of its feed and care. AAC reciprocates with their members by sending them our quarterly newsletter, delicious milk sweets, and photos of our bovine beauties.

Ox Power Alternative Energy Club
9B Stetson St. Brunswick, ME 0401, (207) 725-1047

The Ox Power Alternative Energy Club seeks to fulfill the instructions of Bhaktivedanta Swami Prabhupada regarding the development of ox-powered agriculture and cow protection as the economic basis for a spiritual society. The goal of the Club is to promote the development of small-scale, localized, sustainable agriculture. Membership is available for $15/year.

Lega Anti Vivisezione (Anti Vivisection League)

LAV is a non-violent organization acting in defense of all living beings for their health and respect through research, legislation, dissemination of educational materials, and direct intervention. It is the biggest antivivisection/animal rights organization in Italy and one of the most important ones in all of Europe. Originally founded in 1977, starting in 1980 LAV widened its scope to include animal rights but still kept vivisection in the front lines, due to its anti-scientific nature. Recently, LAV has sponsored EAR, Europe for Animal Rights, an agreement between like-minded national organizations, campaigning in their respective countries for the needs, well-being and vital interests of non-human animals through non-violent, direct and legal action and education and by promoting the ethics and life style (i.e. vegetarianism) of the animal rights movement in Europe, which is dedicated to justice beyond the human species border. LAV and other organizations that join EAR are dedicated to making the world a better place to live for human as well as non-human animal.

LAV, Via Santamaura 72, Roma 00192 ITALY
Tel.0039-6-3973-3292, Fax 6-3973-3462, E-mail: lav@ mclink.it
http://www.mclink.it/assoc/lav

GAIA (Global Action in the Interest of Animals), 169 Av. Princesse Elisabeth, 1030 Brussels, Belgium, Tel. 0032-2-245-2950, Fax 2-215-0943

EFAP (Greek Anti Hunting Initiative), P.O. Box 30736, 10033 Athens, Greece, Tel.0030-1-8948-086, Fax 1-897-3799

AEQUALIS, 12, Rue du Fiez, 92100 Boulogne Billancourt, France, Tel.0033-1-46210803 Fax 1-4621-4498

This recipe, a classic from Italian cuisine, is given by Gianluca Felicetti and Adolfo Sansolini, the dynamic directors of LAV.

RICE STUFFED TOMATOES

4 big round tomatoes	some basil leaves
4 spoonfuls of rice	one cup of olive oil
garlic, one clove	oregano
a small bunch of parsley	salt and pepper to taste

Cut the tomatoes to obtain a cap that will cover the filling. Empty them out, set aside the tomatoes' pulp, sprinkle the inside with salt, pepper and a little olive oil. In a bowl, mix the uncooked rice with finely minced parsley and basil, plus the crushed garlic clove (that will be removed after, its function being only to impart flavor to the mix), one pinch of oregano, a few spoonfuls of olive oil and the tomatoes' inside.

After amalgamating the ingredients, remove the garlic, and stuff the four tomatoes with it. Then top with the tomatoes' "cap". Place the tomatoes in an oiled oven tray, placing big slices of potatoes in between them. Pour abundant olive oil on them and cook in the oven for about 45 minutes.   Serve hot as a side dish, or cold as an entree.

North American Vegetarian Society
P.O. Box 72, Dolgeville, NY 13329

Founded in 1974, the North American Vegetarian Society is a non-profit educational organization dedicated to promoting the vegetarian way of life. Since its inception, NAVS has been affiliated with the International Vegetarian Union. During this time they have organized and sponsored annual vegetarian conferences, including world events. NAVS works year-round to provide factual information to its members, the public, local groups, interested organizations, and the media. Their educational efforts include: publishing *Vegetarian Voice,* a quarterly newsmagazine; sponsoring both regional and national conferences; distributing books and other educational materials by mail and at local and national events; and responding to inquires from all sectors of society. As originator and organizer of the annual celebration of World Vegetarian Day (October 1), NAVS seeks to promote the joy, compassion and life-enhancing possibilities of vegetarianism.

SPANISH RICE

4 stalks celery, diced	1 tsp. salt
1 onion, chopped	1/2 tsp. oregano
1 green pepper, diced	1 tsp. basil
2 cloves garlic	1/4 tsp. paprika
1 tbs. vegetable oil	1 cup chopped tomatoes
1 tsp. chili powder	3 cups warm cooked brown
1 tsp. cumin	rice

Sauté celery, onion, pepper and garlic in oil until vegetables are tender. Add chili powder, cumin, salt, oregano, basil, paprika and tomatoes. Cook until tomatoes are soft. Stir in rice.

PETA—People for the Ethical Treatment of Animals
PETA, P.O. BOX 42516, Washington DC 20015, (301) 770-PETA

"Without movements for social change, we would still have: legalized slavery, child labor, no voting rights for women, segregation, and involuntary human experiments. We can raise our collective voices to change the situation for animals, too. You can start by adopting this motto: *Animals are not ours to eat, wear, experiment on, or use for entertainment.* To find out more, write to PETA's Literature Department.
—Alex Pacheco, Chairman; Ingrid E. Newkirk, National Director

PETA is a national, nonprofit organization, dedicated to establishing the rights and improving the lives of all animals.

MAGICAL MYSTERY TACOS

Who needs beef? Your family will want to eat this delicious makeover of a south-of-the-border classic eight days a week.

1/2 onion, chopped
2 garlic cloves, crushed
1 small bell pepper, diced
1 tbs. vegetable oil
1 tbs. soy sauce
1/2 lb. firm tofu, crumbled

1 tbs. chili powder
1/4 tsp. ground cumin
1/4 tsp. dried oregano
6 corn tortillas or ready-to-eat
   taco shells

Sauté the onion, garlic and bell pepper in oil for 2 or 3 minutes. Add tofu, chili powder, cumin, oregano and soy sauce. Cook for 3 minutes. Add tomato sauce and simmer over low heat until mixture is fairly dry. Heat tortillas in a heavy, ungreased skillet, turning each from side to side until soft and pliable. (Omit this step if using taco shells.) Place a small amount of the tofu mixture in the center, fold the tortilla in half, and remove from heat. Garnish with chopped lettuce, onions, tomatoes, salsa and avocado.

Return To Eden
Vegetarian Supermarket

RTE is owned and operated by Jodi, Wendy and Alan Purcell. In August 1992, when Alan was diagnosed with colon cancer and two uncles who also worked within the family business died of cancer that same year, he agreed with his wife it was time for a change but was not sure of a direction. At home while recovering from surgery and going through chemotherapy, daily news reports illustrated the dangers of chemicals in our food supply and the dangers we incur eating convenience foods. In April of 1993, with no retail grocery experience, Wendy and Alan started researching the natural foods industry— visiting every store in metro Atlanta, working with distributors, and talking to shoppers to find out their shopping needs. In July, with a location acquired, their daughter Jodi joined in the business venture to complete the threesome. For the next six weeks, a massive undertaking was performed by everyone to open by September 1, 1993. Finally, September 1st arrived and RTE opened its doors. With the transformation completed, all involved thought it would be downhill from there, but the work had just started. As each month passed, the Purcells acquired more knowledge and understanding of their customers' needs and desires. The hundred hour weeks were dismissed by the feeling of doing something of great benefit for their fellow man. In November of 1994, Bovine Gelatin Caps were totally removed from the shelves—RTE became TOTALLY VEGETARIAN and CRUELTY FREE. RTE has the distinction of being one of four TOTALLY VEGETARIAN SUPERMARKETS in the U.S. with 7,000 square feet of selling space, displaying over 10,000 items and giving the avid and the novice shopper the most varied choice of products available anywhere. RTE offers the largest selection anywhere of all-natural foods, vitamins, supplement, homeopathy, health & beauty care, and organic produce. Located in Atlanta at 2335 Cheshire Bridge Road, just two blocks east of 1-85. Phone 404/320-EDEN.

VEGAN QUICHE

1 container Vegie Kaas Vegan Cheese Spread
1 Mori Nu soft Tofu
1 cup Westsoy Unsweetened Soy Milk
1 tsp. Bioforce Herbmare
1 tsp. coarse ground black pepper
4 tbs. Ener G Egg Replacer

4 tbs. Lightlife Fakin'Bacon Bits
1 bunch organic baby spinach, rinsed and drained
1/4 large organic red onion, chopped
Soymage Parmesan
1 Maple Lane Wheat-Free Rye Pie Crust

Cream Vegie Kaas Spread and Tofu over low flame, add soy milk, and continue stirring (will look somewhat granular). Add remaining ingredients. Turn into pie crust and sprinkle Soymage Parmesan over top. Bake at 350° degrees for 45 minutes or until firm to touch. Makes 6 wedges.

San Francisco Vegetarian Society
1450 Broadway #4, San Francisco CA 94109

The SFVS is one of the oldest vegetarian groups in the U.S., founded in October 1968. The recipes are given by the dynamic president, Dixie Mahy, vegetarian since 1957.

VEGETABLE ENCHILADAS

Sauté in 1/4 cup oil or water 4 cups mixed diced vegetables (mushroom, onions, bell pepper and celery, all or any).
1 tsp. cumin

1 tsp. salt or vegetable salt
When vegetables start to become transparent, add
1/4 cup sesame seeds
1 small chopped olives
soy cheese (optional)

When mixture is thoroughly warm, fill 4 tortillas and roll them into enchiladas. Bake or fry until tortillas are golden brown. Top with generous amounts of avocado sauce.

In blender mix 1 large avocado, plus:
4 cloves garlic
1 tbs. vegetable oil
1/2 tsp. salt
1/4 water

Serve chilled over enchiladas. The sauce can also be used for vegetables and salad.

━━━━━━━

Sevananda Natural Foods Cooperative
1111 Euclid Ave. NE
Atlanta, GA 30307, (404) 681-2831

Sevananda Community Owned Natural Foods is the Southeast's largest consumer-owned cooperative. For over 20 years, Sevananda has provided the Atlanta area with high quality natural and organic foods. Located in the heart of Little 5 Points, Sevananda offers the finest selection of bulk herbs and spices, local and organic produce, vitamins and supplements, and natural food groceries. Sevananda offers ongoing health, cooking and nutrition classes and a variety of information brochures on healthy living. They avoid purchasing from companies that disregard human rights and environmental health. Sevananda gives preference to local suppliers, producers and growers, and those who demonstrate humane and non-exploitative business practices. They exclude from their product line:

a) products containing artificial chemicals or genetically-engineered foods, or that have been subject to irradiation;
b) products that contain refined sugar, other than fructose in sodas;
c) all animal flesh or animal by-products for which the animal must be slaughtered including beef, fowl, and fish; and
d) soaps and cosmetics that have been developed using cruel and abusive animal laboratory tests.

Sevananda's mission is to empower the community to improve its health and well-being. They accomplish this mission through:

a) facilitating the democratic participation of the members;
b) providing natural and organic foods, and other environmentally sound products, to the Atlanta area and beyond;
c) providing education on cooperative principles, personal health, environmental conservation and consumer issues; and
d) establishing beneficial relationships with the local community and the global cooperative movement.

Sevananda is a consumer-owned cooperative. That means that we are owned by the people who shop here, rather than one person or a select group of investors. You don't have to be a member to shop at Sevananda, but members participate in the business in a special way.

This recipe was developed by Sevananda's Kitchen Manager, John Koch.

RICE SALAD

3 cups cooked rice	1/4 cup red bell
1/4 cup roasted cashews	2 oz. curry vinaigrette
1/4 cup carrots	2 oz. sesame vinaigrette
1/4 cup celery	1/4 tsp. fresh ginger
1/2 cup peas	pinch turmeric
1 scallion	

Combine all ingredients well. You can serve immediately, although allowing the salad to sit for an hour will allow the flavors to develop. You can also refrigerate and serve chilled.

The vegetarian wave is spreading all over the African continent. Lately, new vegetarian societies are being formed where none existed before, and they need reading material. Those who can send vegetarian magazines, books and other literature (preferably in English) should write Maxwell G. Lee, Hon. General Secretary, International Vegetarian Union, 10 King's Drive, Marple, Stockport, Cheshire, SK6 6NQ, England, United Kingdom, phone/ fax 0044-0161-4275850; or e-mail 100754.1763@compuserve.com.

Vegetarian Awareness Network

VEGETARIAN AWARENESS NETWORK / VEGANET is an all-volunteer, non-sectarian, nonpartisan, not-for profit, educational, social service organization. VEGANET networks nationally with consumers, communities and companies: to encourage eco-friendliness, kindness and healthfulness for products, people and the planet through informed eating; to advance public awareness of the benefits of a vegetarian life style; to assist consumers in making informed dietary decisions; to enhance the visibility and accessibility of vegetarian products and services; to facilitate the formation and expansion of local vegetarian organizations; to promote healthful living, environmental healing, and respect for all life. The NETWORK is the originator and sponsor of Vegetarian Awareness Month, a nationwide event celebrated annually in October. They also have a speaker's

bureau; research library; and a co-op mail packet for consumers—
VEGEKIT. Information and referral services. Founded 1980.

National Headquarters 202-347-VEGE, PO Box 3545,
Washington, DC 20007
Communications Center 423-558-VEGE, PO Box 321, Knoxville,
TN 37901. Toll-free link line: 1-800-EAT-VEGE

The enclosed recipe was sent to VAN by Brad Wolff, president of
Vegan Foods in Memphis, TN.

HOLIDAY PUMPKIN STEW

Pumpkin Stew is a wonderful main course for Holiday Season
celebrations. Served in the pumpkin itself, it is a very attractive center-
piece and is a healthy and humane alternative to turkey or ham.

**1 large pumpkin that is wider
   than it is tall, and will stand
   upright.
2 cups dried navy beans,
   soaked overnight in 5 cups
   water, then drained
2 medium yellow onions, diced
1 large clove garlic, minced
2 tbs. olive oil or 1/2 cup
   water
3 cups fresh corn cut off the
   cob or 3 cups frozen corn**

**6 large, ripe, fresh tomatoes,
   peeled and stewed
1 tbs. dried or 2 Tbs. fresh
   oregano
1 tbs. dried or 2 Tbs. fresh
   basil
2 bay leaves
1/2 tsp. black pepper or to
   taste
1 tsp. dried or 2 tsp. fresh
   marjoram
1 tsp. salt, or to taste**

To prepare pumpkin: cut top from pumpkin and scoop out seeds and
stringy fibers. Replace top, put on cookie sheet in a 325 degree oven
for 30 minutes (or microwave on high 15 minutes) until somewhat tender. With a large spoon, scrape out pulp to equal 4 cups when diced,
being careful to leave at least an inch on the sides, so the pumpkin will
stand up.
    To prepare stew: Sauté onions and garlic until tender in 2 tbs. olive
oil or 1/2 cup water in a 5 quart heavy pot. Put soaked and drained

navy beans, diced pumpkin and seasoning (except salt) in pot with
enough water to cover about 2 inches the above ingredients. Bring to
a boil, then turn heat to low, cover and simmer, stirring occasionally,
for 2 hours or until beans are tender. Add tomatoes, corn and salt.
Bring to a boil, then turn down to a simmer for 30 minutes more.

WHEN READY TO SERVE: place pumpkin shell on serving
plate and ladle hot stew into it.

Vegetarians International:Feeding People With Love Worldwide
P.O. Box 45, Badger, California 93603

Vegetarians International is a cultural movement promoting vegetarianism, spirituality and distribution of free vegetarian food to needy
people. The world needs a new ethic and we believe that spiritual
vegetarianism is the fastest and safest way to global improvement.

A gentle, nonsectarian but powerful network is growing, day after
day, working to bring progressive positive changes in the United
States and all over the world. Its members are moving from the old
stereotype "American Dream" to a new enlightened vision, a new
paradigm of love, knowledge and respect for life.

In the near future people should be able to grow their own food,
heal their own body and choose freely their spiritual path. The end of
the Cold War, an artificial situation created to scare and control the
masses, has joyfully accelerated this amazing transformation.

Our goal is to educate people about their eating habits and eliminate hunger all over the world, encouraging and promoting free vegetarian food distribution. Vegetarianism is not an event or a temporary
fashion but the most natural, honest and sincere way to feed your
human body. We, Vegetarians International, are on the front lines of
this Global Renaissance that is touching the hearts and minds of
millions.

Many experts on social change are trying to understand and define
what is happening now. Post-industrialist Alvin Toffler calls it Third
Wave; futurist Hazel Henderson, the Solar Age. John Naisbitt speaks
of the Information Age in the Global Village, predicted by the media-

prophet, Marshall McLuhan. Physicist Fritjof Capra describes this historical time as the Turning Point.

Astrologers predicted this period to be the dawn of a new age of Aquarius, a time of joyful and long-lasting happiness. More than 500 hundred years ago, the last avatar of Lord Krishna, Sri Caitanya Mahaprabhu, appeared in Bengal and predicted the rise of Golden Age—soon, people all over the world will become vegetarian and chant the names of God, dancing in ecstasy in the streets of every town and village.

Nobel Prize winner Isaac Bashevis Singer explained that "vegetarianism" is his strong, radical statement against the dysfunctionality of the world. Brother Ron Pickarski, a Franciscan monk, following the example and the compassionate teachings of St. Francis of Assisi, the patron saint of animals and ecology, proclaimed that "When people learn to love themselves and their fellow human beings, then and only then will vegetarianism predominate the universe. And the funny thing is, they will not perceive it as vegetarianism, just simply loving."

The famous pacifist and civil rights leader Dick Gregory, in a 1979 interview, foresaw that "Vegetarianism will definitely become a PEOPLE'S MOVEMENT." Corporate trend-spotter Faith Popcorn didn't hesitate to say that "The future is vegetarian!" The *Diet for a New America*, according to John Robbins, is totally vegetarian. Vegetarianism is not only a time of history that comes and goes—it is a peaceful state of mind, an ancient and new life style. It is the Garden of Eden.

The poet Gary Snyder wrote that a Great Subculture, whose roots stretch back in very ancient times, is spreading now all over the world. We call this period of awakening and positive transformation not just "Sub" but, rather, the Real Age of Humanity.

A fundamental shift in everyone's consciousness will make the difference—everywhere, people are expressing a new, much needed, love for the Absolute Truth, for God the Father and God the Mother, a new compassionate respect for all living creatures, the real inspiring alternative to the violent dominant culture of slaughterhouses and meat eating.

This New Compassionate Renaissance reveals finer spiritual approaches, fruitful values and clear understanding, a return to remembrance and appreciation of the lost brotherhood and sisterhood of humankind. Our goal is to favor the spontaneous rising of groups, willing to stop the bad karma of killing animals for food.

No doubt we are approaching a major turning point in human history. To free society we have to abolish the last, great authorized crime: animal slavery. For many centuries human slavery was justified by politicians and religious leaders. It was called a "Divine Institution" and a "Moral Relation"—not immoral, but God's institution. The slave trade was openly accepted in the public market, recognized as legitimate, blessed in accordance with civilized humane principles and the holy laws of established revealed religions.

People are trying to use this same justification for animal torture, but too many intelligent and sensitive persons are perceiving the present transformative changes which will lead toward the realization of a new civilization, so much hoped for in every previous era. We are very close, it will happen in a short time. It will be the first peaceful, global revolution of history. The VEGETARIAN REVOLUTION stops the killing and teaches love and respect for all life. Now, please meditate with us for a moment on this new and exciting FUTURE VISION: What would this Earth Planet be like if people were able to stop meat eating and discover their full potential? Remember that your love, your compassion and your creative imagination are absolutely needed to generate soon such a wonderful epoch. We are all interconnected—God, angels, humans, animals, plants and even beings living on other planets.

The third millennium is coming soon and can be an irresistible and attractive experience for all of us. It is not a dream, a mirage or a new age utopia—we are speaking about something real and possible, a new and blissful society where any kind of killing is just an old, cruel memory of a past uncivilized culture.

Don't look at the sky waiting for the "manna" to come down. Be spiritual, take responsibility here and now, look around in the streets, recognize your brothers and sisters and share with love your "daily bread".

Be part of the VEGETARIAN REVOLUTION!
Love, respect and celebrate ALL LIFE!
God will bless you!

RHUBARB SUPRISE PUDDING

4 cups sliced rhubarb
3/4 cup flour
1 tsp. baking powder
1/2 cup rolled oats
1 1/2 cups sugar

1/4 cup butter
1/2 cup milk
1 tbs. corn flour
1/2 cup boiling water pinch
   salt

Wash the rhubarb and cut into 1/2 inch to 1 inch slices. Spread evenly in the bottom of a greased casserole dish. Sift together flour, baking powder and salt. Add the rolled oats. Melt the butter and blend into it 3/4 cup of sugar. Add this to the dry ingredients, alternating with the milk, mixing well after each addition. Spread over the rhubarb. Combine the remaining 3/4 cup of sugar with the corn flour and a pinch of salt and spread over the batter. Pour boiling water over all. Bake in a moderate oven for about an hour. Serve warm or cold with whipped cream.

The Vegetarian Resource Group
Box 1463, Baltimore, MD 21203 USA

The Vegetarian Resource Group is a non-profit organization aimed to bring healthy changes in schools, workplace and community. Membership is $20. Vegetarian Journal is published bi-monthly and is one of the benefit members enjoy. VRG produces books, brochures and software for consumers, teachers and health professionals.

ASURE

This dessert is made at the same time each year to commemorate a number of important events in Islam. The dish supposedly origi-nated on the day that the Great Flood subsided and Noah and his family were able to go on land again. They collected all the food they had left—mostly dried fruits and nuts—and cooked it in one big pot. Tradition dictates that the dish be shared with at least seven poor neighbors.

1 cup wheat berries (available in health-food stores)
3/4 cup walnuts
1/2 cup hazelnuts
1/2 cup chickpeas
7 dried figs

10 dried apricots
1/2 cup raisins
1 cup sugar or other
sweetener
1/4 cup rose water (optional)
cinnamon to taste

In separate bowls, soak the wheat berries, nuts, and chickpeas for at least eight hours. Rub the chickpeas to loosen as many skins as possible and discard the skins and the water.   Cook chickpeas in fresh water until tender. Drain the wheat and cook covered in about eight cups fresh water until tender. Meanwhile, soak the dried fruit in a little warm water for about 15 minutes, drain and chop. Drain the nuts, rubbing them to remove the hazelnut skins, and chop. Once the wheat berries are cooked, drain off any excess water and reserve. Puree in a food processor.

Combine the wheat berries, fruits, nuts, raisins, sweetener, and the liquid in a large soup pot and simmer uncovered, stirring frequently, for 15 minutes or until mixture becomes more gooey than soupy. Add water if necessary during cooking. Mix in the optional rose water and sprinkle with cinnamon when done. Serve hot or cold. Serves 10.
—from *Vegetarian Journal*, recipe
courtesy of Birsen Davis

The Vegetarian Society of Georgia
P.O. Box 2164, Norcross, Georgia 30091-2164

The Society had its first official meeting in September 1990, and since then has grown up to be one of the largest vegetarian societies in the U.S. We have added a North Georgia Chapter (706/ 782-1556), based in Clayton, and a Southside Chapter (770/ 487-0431) for those who live south of metro Atlanta in the area of Peachtree City, Fayetteville or Tyrone. More chapters are planned throughout the state. We meet monthly, usually for a potluck dinner. We provide speakers for groups and initiated a class "Going Vegetarian" which is taught by members in several metro Atlanta community schools, where we also teach vegetarian cooking classes. VSG members receive a monthly newsletter which is filled with vegetarian-related information.

CARROT CAKE

Preheat oven to 350°

1 cup salad oil	3 cups grated raw carrots
2 cups brown sugar	1 cup chopped nuts - walnuts
1 1/4 cups water or soymilk	or pecans
4 cups unbleached white flour	1 small can crushed pineap-
2 tsp. baking powder	ple, packed in its own juice
2 tsp. baking soda	(drain and measure juice, if
1 tsp. salt	juice in can is less than 1/4
1 1/2 tsp. cinnamon	cup, add enough water or
1/2 tsp. allspice	soymilk to make 1/4 cup)

Blend oil and sugar; add water and beat. Sift the flour with remaining ingredients and add to sugar mixture. Add carrots and nuts and mix well. Bake in 3 oiled and floured layer pans or one 9x13" cake pan at 350° for 35-40 minutes, or until toothpick inserted in center comes out clean (baking time may be less if using small round pans). I used three round layer pans, but only used two of them for the cake.

LEMON FROSTING

**4 cups confectioners' sugar
1 stick margarine, softened
Juice and grated rind of one lemon**

With an electric mixer set at low speed, cream the sugar and margarine. Beat in the lemon juice a little at a time, until you reach the right consistency. Stir in the lemon rind. Frosts one large cake.

Zen Monk
Rochester Zen Center
7 Arnold Park
Rochester, NY 14607

SZECHWAN EGGPLANT AND TOFU

3 tbs. sesame oil	Optional: pinch cayenne
1/3 cup chopped onion	pepper
3 cloves garlic	2 tbs. tamari
3 1/3 cups eggplant, peeled	2/3 cup water
and cubed into 1/2"	1 tsp. rice wine vinegar
squares	1 tsp. maple syrup
1 tsp. grated fresh ginger	2 1/2 tbs. water
1/8 tsp. ground anise	4 tsp. arrowroot powder
1/4 tsp. salt	1 pound tofu cubed
1/8 tsp. pepper	

Heat the oil in a large skillet or wok and sauté the onion and garlic until onion is soft. Add the eggplant, ginger, anise, salt, pepper and cayenne and sauté until eggplant begins to wilt.

Add the tamari, water, vinegar and maple syrup, cover and cook until eggplant is tender, about 15 minutes.

Mix the 2 1/2 tbs. water with the arrowroot powder. Add to the cooking liquid and simmer over low heat until it thickens. Add tofu and cook for 5 minutes. Serve hot. Serves 4-6.

This recipe has been excerpted from *Food for the Gods: Vegetarianism and the World's Religions* by Rynn Berry, Pythagorean Publishers, PO Box 8174, JAF Stn. New York NY 10016.

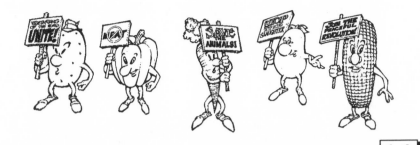

11

Recipes of Vegetarian Restaurants

"More people are killed through the stomach than by the sword."
—Seneca, Roman Philosopher (4 B.C. - A.D. 65)

Vegetarian Poll

In a 1991 Gallup Poll, conducted for the National Restaurant Association, about 30 percent of respondents said they look for a restaurant with vegetarian items when they eat out.

Atlanta, Georgia
Cafe Sunflower, 5975 Roswell Road, Suite 353, Atlanta, GA 30328
(404)256-1675

"Our goal is to serve you delicious, healthful meals that draw from Asian, Southwestern and European cuisine, in an elegant and smoke-free environment. Most of our recipes are vegan, and prepared with-

193

out any animal products; others make light use of cheese and milk. The following services are also available—carry out, catering, parties."

CHOCOLATE CAKE

3 cups all purpose flour (not Gold Medal), can substitute one cup bread flour for one of the all purpose.
2 tsp. baking soda
1/2 tsp. salt
3/4 cup cocoa

3/4 cup (1 1/2 sticks) margarine, softened
2 cups sugar
1/4 water
1 1/4 cups soy milk combined with 1/2 cup water
1 tsp. vanilla

Combine dry ingredients and set aside. Cream margarine. Gradually add sugar. Add 1/4 cup water and beat well. Add dry mixture alternately with soy milk/water mixture, beginning and ending with dry mixture. Add vanilla. Turn up mixer, speed and beat well for about 5 minutes. Divide batter between two oiled and floured 9-inch round pans. Bake at 350° F for 30-40 minutes or until toothpick inserted in center comes out clean.

Icing:
8 tbs. (1 stick) margarine, softened

4 cups powdered sugar
6 Tbs. cocoa powder
soy milk

Cream margarine. Gradually add 2 cups powdered sugar and all of cocoa powder. Mix in 1-2 tbs. soy milk. Gradually add remainder of powdered sugar and enough soy milk
    (1 tbs. at a time) to create desired consistency. I cut off tops of cake layers and freeze separately before icing. It makes them easier to work with.

———————

Christchurch, New Zealand
Gopal's Vegetarian Restaurant, 143 Worcester St., Christchurch, New Zealand, Phone 011 649 303-4885 (from the U.S.)

KIWI FRUIT CHUTNEY

4 cups kiwi fruit, peeled and
  diced
1 cup raw sugar
1/2 cup dried currants
2-3 green chilies minced

1 Tbs. ghee or vegetable oil
1/2 tsp. fennel seeds
2 sticks of cinnamon
1 tsp. of chopped fresh mint
1 Tbs. grated fresh ginger

Heat the ghee or oil in the pot. Add fresh chilies together with fennel seeds, cinnamon bark and grated ginger. Fry spices on medium flame, stir with wooden spoon, until lightly brown. Add diced kiwi fruit. Stir fry for about 5 minutes. Add sugar and dried currants. Let sugar dissolve. On low flame simmer for about 15 minutes until kiwi fruit is jam-like consistency. Stir occasionally. Add fresh herbs at the end.

═══════════════

Florence, Italy
Sedano Allegro, Borgo la Croce 20 rosso, Firenze 50121 Italy

This restaurant, right in the historical center of Florence, is managed by Chef Virgilio Potini and his family. Here you can enjoy the taste of Italian cuisine and the warm hospitality of an Italian family.

CALZONE

Dough:
2 tbs. yeast
1 cup warm water (105° F)
1 tsp. salt
1/3 cup oil (not olive oil)
2 cups flour
oil for deep frying

Filling:
1/ cup chopped mozzarella
  cheese
1/2 cup Parmesan cheese
1 1/2 cups ricotta cheese
1/3 cup chopped parsley
1 cup deep fried eggplant
  cubes
2 tsp. salt
1 tsp. pepper
1/4 tsp. hing (asafetida)

Add yeast to warm water and let sit for 1 minute. Add salt, oil, and flour. Knead for 3 minutes. Sprinkle tabletop with flour. Separate dough into 2-inch balls. Cover with damp cloth and let them rise for 45 minutes. While dough is rising, mix all the filling ingredients together. Heat oil in wok until very hot.

Roll out balls into 6-inch circles. Divide stuffing into 8 portions. Place stuffings in center and fold over. Place fork in flour and use to seal edges. Fry in hot oil for about 1 minute on each side until they are reddish brown. Serve hot. Makes 8.

Los Angeles, California
Govinda's Dining Club, 3764 Watseka Avenue, Los Angeles 90034

DELUXE TOFU SANDWICH WITH CORN CHIPS

Sandwich: (one)

firm Tofu (Bean Curd) 1/4 lb.	**sour cream**
ghee oil	**sprouts**
soy sauce	**mustard**
rennet-free cheese	**ketchup**
lettuce	**water**
sliced tomatoes	**2 slices of your favorite bread**

Cut tofu into 4 half-inch wide rectangles by cutting the block of tofu on its end. Heat ghee or oil in pan until near smoking. Fry tofu strips until golden brown. Take out strips and drain. Put into container with 50% water and 50% soy sauce. Cover and soak for approximately one hour. Take two slices of your favorite bread, coat one side with ketchup and the other side with mustard. (Toast if preferred.) Layer tofu, lettuce, cheese, tomatoes, sprouts and sour cream to taste.

Corn Chips:	**ghee or oil**
Corn tortillas	**soy sauce**

Take corn tortillas and cut into eight pieces—like a pizza. Fry in hot ghee or oil until golden brown. Remove, drain and spray with soy sauce.

Los Angeles Smog

"A recent study by California Institute of Technology atmospheric chemist Glen Cass has found that in the eternal summer of laid-back Los Angeles, the single greatest source of the city's legendary smog is not jets or cigarettes or car exhaust, but charred meat from backyard cook-outs and restaurant grills."

> —from *Vegetarian News*, newsletter of the Vegetarian Society Inc.

Melbourne, Australia
Gopal's, 139 Swanston St., Melbourne, Victoria 3000 Australia
Phone 011 613 650-1578

BAKED STUFFED AVOCADOS

In this succulent and unusual entree, avocados are stuffed with tofu and green peas, smothered in a lemon-chili-coconut sauce, and baked.
Preparation time: 10 minutes. Cooking time: 10 minutes. Baking time: 10 minutes.

2 large, firm but ripe avocados
2 tbs. (40 ml) olive oil
1/4 tsp. (1 ml) yellow asafetida powder
1 tsp. (5 ml) chopped fresh ginger
1 cup (250 ml) firm tofu, diced to 1.25 cm (1/2 inch) cubes
1 tsp. (5 ml) Chinese sesame oil

1 tbs. (20 ml) sweet soy sauce
1 match-box size chunk of creamed coconut, chopped
1/2 cup (125 ml) cooked green peas
1 tbs. (20 ml) fresh lemon juice
1 tsp. (5 ml) salt
1 tbs. (20 ml) minced fresh coriander leaves

1) Carefully run a knife from the stem end downwards and right around the avocados. Twist to separate the two halves. Remove the seeds.

2) With a spoon, scoop out the avocado flesh leaving a 1.25 cm (1/2 inch) border. Chop the avocado flesh into large rough chunks.

3) Heat the olive oil in a heavy non-stick frying pan over medium heat. Add the asafetida and sauté for a few seconds. Add the ginger and sauté for 1 minute. Add the tofu and stir fry carefully. When the tofu is browned, drizzle on the sesame oil, chili sauce, and soy sauce. Fold in the creamed coconut, stirring until it melts.

4) Add the peas, lemon juice, salt, minced fresh coriander, and stir well. Finally, add the avocado pieces, stir to mix, and remove from the heat. Place the avocado halves carefully on a flame-proof gratin dish and add the stuffing. Bake in a preheated oven at 180 C / 355 F for 10 minutes and serve immediately. Serves 4.

New York, New York
Caravan of Dreams, 405 East 6th Street, New York NY 10009

This restaurant, managed by Angel Moreno Segura, specializes in creating light dishes. All fruits, vegetables and grains are organically grown.

VEGETARIAN SPANISH STEW
POTAJEMADRILENO VEGETARIANO

1 lb. dried chickpeas (washed
  and soaked overnight with
  1 tbs. of sea salt in tepid
  filtered water)
2 lb.. fresh spinach (leaves
  only)
6 tbs. virgin olive oil
1 bay leaf

1/2 small garlic head
1 plump garlic clove
1 level tsp. paprika
1 fresh sprig of parsley
1 large tomato, diced
1 tbs. whole wheat or spelt
  flour (wheat free)
1 tbs. sea salt

Discard the water from the soaked chickpeas. In a 6 qt. heavy-bottomed stockpot, heat (but not boil) 2-3 qt. of filtered water. Add the chickpeas, 1/2 whole head of garlic, one bay leaf and one small peeled whole onion. Cover, and let it simmer for 2 1/2 to 3 hours at low medium heat. Cut the spinach leaves into small pieces, add them to the stockpot, and let them cook for 15 more minutes. Heat the oil in a frying pan. Dice and add the remaining onion, and sauté for 10 minutes to a light golden color. Then add the diced tomato. Shortly after, add the flour and stir. Finally, add the paprika, sauté with the rest for a few minutes, and quickly remove from the heat to avoid losing vitamins. Puree this mix into a sauce in a food mill, food processor, or blender. Pour the sauce over the chickpeas and season with salt to taste. Crush the parsley with the garlic clove in a mortar with a pestle. Gradually add one tbs. of the chickpea stock, mixing it together. Add this mix back to the chickpea stock and let it all cook together for 15 more minutes. Enjoy and buen provecho. Serves 6.

Paris, France
A La Ville de Jagannath, 101 Rue St. Maur, Paris 75011 France

ALMOND STUDDED KOFTA BALLS
WITH A VELVET RED TOMATO SAUCE

1/2 medium sized white
 cabbage
1/2 cup coarsely chopped
 almonds
1/2 cup coarsely chopped
 cilantro
1 inch of peeled ginger, finely
 minced
1 tsp. of ground turmeric
1 tsp. of freshly ground
 coriander seeds
1/2 tsp. of garam masala
1/4 tsp. of paprika

1/4 tsp. of fennel seeds
1 cup of sifted chick pea flour
3/4 tsp. of baking powder
1 1/2 tsp. of sea salt or to taste
ghee for deep frying

Ingredients for the sauce:
1 tbs. of ghee
1 inch stick of cinnamon
1/2 inch piece of ginger peeled
 and minced
1 tsp. of cumin seeds
1/2 tsp. of black mustard seeds

1/8 tsp. asafetida
5 fresh curry leaves
1/2 tsp. turmeric
8 medium sized tomatoes,
   pealed and chopped

1 tbs. of jaggery, raw cane
   sugar
1 1/2 tsp. salt or to taste
1/2 tsp. garam masala
chopped fresh cilantro for
   garnishing

Wash and core a fresh 1/2 white cabbage. With a large knife, cut into cubes that can easily fit into a food processor. Process for about 5-8 seconds or until you have an even mix with no large pieces of cabbage left. Remove from the processor and with your hands squeeze out as much of the excess juice as you can, placing it in a mixing bowl. Now you can add to this your chopped almonds, cilantro, ginger, turmeric, coriander, garam masala, paprika, fennel seeds—mixing well.

Now put a tablespoon of ghee in a heavy bottomed sauce pot and heat over a medium flame until the ghee is hot but not burning, then add quickly the ginger cinnamon, cumin seeds, mustard seeds, until the cumin seeds begin to splutter and turn gray (I recommend an antisplatter screen). Then add the asafetida, fresh curry leaves, immediately followed by the chopped peeled tomatoes.

Raise the heat to high and add the turmeric jaggery and salt. When the sauce comes to a boil, reduce the heat and simmer until you have a smooth sauce (about 15-20 minutes).

Place a deep frying pan with your ghee (or vegetable oil) on a medium heat. While it is heating, you can finish your kofta mix. Mix your sifted chickpea flour, baking powder and salt and add to your cabbage mix. This must be done just before frying; if not, the salt makes the cabbage bleed and you finish with a messy mush. Mix well and with your hands form small balls about 3/4 inch in diameter and put them to the side. When your ghee is hot but not smoking, gently place the balls in it—not too many at a time or else your koftas will be greasy. Fry until they are a deep golden brown, taking them out with a slotted spoon and letting them drain on paper towels. Fry the next batchs until you have no more mix. Now add the garam masala to your sauce.

Place the balls, 2 or 3 per person, on a plate and pour the sauce over it, garnishing it with some freshly chopped cilantro. Offer this to someone you love. Serves 6-7 people.

Rome, Italy
Margutta Vegetariano Ristorante, Via Margutta 118
Rome, Italy 00187, tel. 06-3-265-0577

Established in 1980 by Claudio Vannini, this restaurant has been known as the most elegant and famous vegetarian restaurant in Italy. Attractive for its excellent cuisine, the filmmaker Federico Fellini and actor Marcello Mastrianni helped make this place a stylish favorite of Italian film stars and TV personalities.

TAGLIOLINI IN HOT AND SOUR SAUCE

1 kilo San Marzano tomatoes
  (green and long-shaped)
1 clove garlic
1 hot chili
1 small bunch basil

30 grams pine nuts
20 grams parmesan cheese
3 tbs. extra virgin olive oil
salt to taste

Chop garlic very fine and chop pine nuts. Pour both in a large pan with oil and chili.
    Slice the tomatoes lengthwise into long, thin pieces and stir into the pan. I suggest to use very green, hard tomatoes. Then add salt, and basil finely minced.
    Cook the pasta separately by pouring it in abundant salty boiling water. Drain the pasta and add in the sauce. Allow to cook for a short while, then mix in the grated parmesan. Serves 4.

San Diego, California
Second Nature Vegetarian Cafe, 4652 Mission Blvd.
Pacific Beach, CA 92109, (619) 272-7399

"We aim to be a fun, casual meeting place where fresh, healthy, delicious food is offered at reasonable prices. We believe in treating our customers with kindness, respect and flexibility.

Also, Second Nature strives to promote vegetarianism, holistic health, human rights, animal rights, environmentalism through awareness, education and by example. We are committed to feeding the homeless, recycling extensively, and otherwise supporting worthy causes. We hire fun, free-thinking individuals, and provide them with love, support and a progressive work environment. Through its daily activities, Second Nature also seeks to embody the higher values of respect, creativity, generosity, faith, trust and love. In these ways, we hope to touch the world."

BANANA CAROB CHIP CAKE

In a small bowl, mix maple syrup, vegetable oil, egg replacer powder and bananas together. In another bowl, mix flour, baking soda and carob chips. Mix together, using about 30 strokes. Spoon into tube pan or two round cake pans and bake at 350 degrees for about 40 minutes, or until skewer inserted in center of cake comes out clean. Yield: 12 large slices.

San Francisco, California
Millennium, 246 McAllister Street, San Francisco 94102
tel.(415) 487-9800, Manager: Margaret Malone

The philosophy of the Millennium Restaurant favors healthy living, serving organic cuisine and supporting sustainable agriculture and local produce suppliers.

QUINOA-CORN VERA CRUZ

This is a one pan, quick and easy main dish. You can also use this recipe as a filling for crepes. Top the crepes with a tomatillo sauce and you have created an elegant brunch or dinner entree. You can also use corn tortillas instead of the crepes for a more rustic entree.

1/2 cup of vegetable broth or water
1 large onion, diced

3 cloves garlic, diced
1 medium red or green bell pepper

3 medium ripe tomatoes
1/4 tsp. cayenne
2 ears yellow corn, kernels
   removed about 1 cup
1/2 cup frozen green peas
   (blanched quickly)
1 16 oz can red kidney beans,
   drained

2 cups cooked quinoa and
   millet mixed together or
   other cooked grain
1/2 cup fresh basil leaves,
   roughly chopped
2 tablespoons fresh marjoram
   or other fresh herb
sea salt to taste
pepper to taste

In a large skillet, bring vegetable broth (or water) to a boil. Add the onions, garlic, and red bell pepper. Sauté until onions are translucent, over a high temperature. Add the tomatoes and cayenne, simmer until the tomatoes are tender and the juice has been released. Add the corn, green peas, red kidney beans and simmer for about a minute. Add the quinoa-millet mixture, blend well with the vegetable mixture. Stir in the basil, marjoram, sea salt, and pepper and serve with a mixed green salad.   Serves 4.

━━━━━━━━━━━━━

San Luis Obispo, California
Natural Flavors, 570 Higuera St. #12 , San Luis Obispo CA 93401
(805) 781-9040

Nature provides the flavors, we provide the services. "Our blessings and praise go to all who plant, nurture, harvest, forage, and provide the fruits of our generous, yet fragile bountiful Earth."

KARMAL

1 cup Rice Dream, or water,
   tea etc.
1 cup rice syrup

1/2 cup almond or any other
   nut butter
1/4 salt (optional) or soy sauce

Simmer rice syrup and Rice Dream until caramelized. Add salt and nut butter. Blend thoroughly.

Seattle, Washington
Silence Heart Nest, 5247 University Way NE, Seattle WA 98105
(206) 524-4008

MIXED VEGETABLE CURRY

1/2 lb. onions, chopped
2-3 tsp. fresh ginger chopped
2-3 fresh garlic, chopped
1/2 lb. tomatoes, diced (fresh or canned)
3/4 lb. cauliflower, cut into bite-sized florets
3/4 lb. carrots, peeled and cut into 1" sticks (julienne)
1/2 lb. green peppers, sliced thin

1/3 c frozen peas
2 tbs. canola, peanut or olive oil
1-2 tsp. salt
1 1/2 tbs. spice mix (mix together: 1/4 tsp. cayenne, 1/2 tsp. garam masala, 1 tsp. cumin, 1 tsp. turmeric, 1 tsp. coriander powder, 1 tsp. paprika)

Heat oil over medium heat. When slightly smoky, add onion. Fry until translucent. Then add garlic and fry until slightly golden. Add in ginger and continuously stir so that the mix does not stick to the bottom of the pot. When it turns golden, add the salt and 1 1/2 tbs. of the spice mix. Stir for 2-3 minutes. Add tomatoes and let cook for another 10 minutes. Add carrots; cook another 10 minutes. Then add cauliflower and peppers; cook till done.

Stir often so curry does not stick to the bottom of the pot; cooking time can be expedited by covering pot, although leaving pot open allows a thicker sauce to develop as more water evaporates while cooking.

Quotes from Sri Chinmoy

"The consciousness of food depends mostly on the consciousness of the cook."

"The cleanliness of the surroundings does not immediately or directly affect the food. First it affects the consciousness of the cook. When the cook is affected, then naturally the product will be affected. Cleanliness is of paramount importance, purity is of paramount importance. Everything is of paramount importance from the beginning to the end when you cook. It will also be of considerable help if you can be in meditative consciousness."

Tel Aviv, Israel
Eternity, Ben Yehuda Street, Tel Aviv, Israel

CARROT SUPREME SALAD

16 cups
4-6 cups soy butter
1 cup diced celery
1 cup diced peppers
1 cup relish drained
1 1/2 cups yeast flakes

1/2 cup olive oil
1 tbs. veggie salt
1/2 cup tamari
1 tbs. kelp
1 cup honey

Mix all ingredients well.

Tucson, Arizona
Govinda's, 711 E. Blacklidge Dr., East off of 1st Ave., tel. 792-0630

EGGPLANT MEDALLION

1 firm eggplant sliced in
round 1/4" thick pieces
Make batter from 1 cup
chickpea flour
1 tsp. gr. coriander
1 tsp. cumin powder

3/4 tsp. turmeric
3/4 tsp. asafetida
1/2 tsp. cinnamon
1/4 tsp. cayenne pepper
1/4 tsp. baking soda
1 tsp. sea salt

Sift chickpea flour in bowl, add all spices, slowly wisk cold water until you have a smooth batter thick enough to coat the eggplant. Heat canola or any good quality oil in wok or skillet over medium-high heat. Dip the eggplant slices in batter, then into hot oil, one at a time. Let fry for 2 minutes on each side. Take out and drain in basket on side.

CASHEW PATE´

1/2 cup baked till golden cashew
1/2 cube tofu
1/3 cup canola oil
1/4 cup lemon juice

1/3 bunch fresh parsley
1/4 cup tamari
1/2 tsp. asafetida (hing)
1 tsp. salt

In food processor blend till smooth. In skillet, dry roast 1/3 cup sesame seeds till golden. Add 1/4 tsp. asafetida and 1/4 tsp. sea salt.

Put eggplant medallions on tray. Add spoonful cashew paté. Sprinkle sesame seeds. Add 1 slice of tomato and a few sprouts.

Venice, California
Venus Of Venice, 1202 Abbot Kinney Blvd., Venice CA 90291
(310) 392-1987

"Vegetarianism is one of the main, accessible links toward becoming loving and compassionate toward all living things."
—Venus Michelle Garret

VENUS FRESH-FRUIT COBBLER

Satisfy your sweet tooth naturally with this juicy dessert from the vegetarian restaurant Venus of Venice. Berries or your favorite firm-textured fruits can be substituted for those listed in the recipe.

2 cups walnuts
2 cups almonds
1 1/4 cups raisins
1 1/4 cups pitted dates
1/2 cup pure maple syrup
1/4 cup spring water

2 to 3 ripe mangoes, peeled, thinly sliced
3 ripe kiwi fruit, peeled, thinly sliced
1 medium-size papaya, peeled, thinly sliced

Optional garnishes: raspberries, strawberries, mint leaves.

To make pie crust, using food processor or blender, chop walnuts and almonds (in batches if needed) until of medium coarseness (not too fine). Transfer chopped nuts to mixing bowl. In food processor or blender, combine raisins, dates, syrup and water; process until blended and smooth. Stir raisin mixture into chopped nuts until well mixed. Into canola-oiled 9 inch pie plate or 9 by 12 inch baking pan, spread crust along bottom and up sides of pan. On pie crust bottom, arrange a layer of mangoes; add a layer of kiwi, then of papaya. Garnish as desired with berries. Slice or spoon onto plates. Makes 12 servings.

Per serving: 437 calories, 9 grams protein, 24 grams, 55 grams carbohydrate, 10 milligrams sodium, 0 milligrams cholesterol.

━━━━━━━━━

Washington D.C.
Soul Vegetarian Cafe, 2606 Georgia Ave. NW, Washington D.C. 2000

NORTHEAST AFRICAN MILLET PATTIES

3 cups cooked millet (a tiny, round golden grain that becomes light and fluffy when cooked, popular in India and China). To cook millet, bring 2 1/2 cups water to a boil. Add 1 cup millet, cover and simmer over medium heat 15 minutes. Remove from heat; let sit uncovered 20 minutes. Makes about 3 cups.
1/2 cup nut butter such as cashew, almond, peanut or tahini
1 tbs. onion powder
1 tbs. tamari
1 tsp. celery seed
1 tbs. canola oil

Mix all ingredients together. Form into patties; brown on both sides in lightly oiled skillet. Makes 6 patties.

Per serving: 296 calories; 10 grams protein; 14 grams fat; 34 grams carb; 0 chol; 176 mg sod; 3 grams fiber.

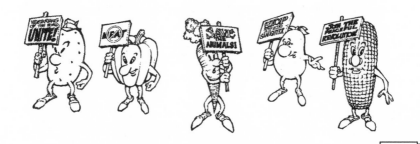

12

Recipes from
Vegetarian Cookbooks

"We are the new wave of vegetarian cooking, we believe in world peace through the power of the fork."

> —Tanya Petrovna of the vegetarian
> restaurant Native Foods, Smoke Tree Village,
> 1775 E. Palm Canyon Drive, Palm Springs,
> CA (619)416-0070

Ayurvedic Cooking For Self Healing
by Usha Lad & Vasant Lad, The Ayurvedic Press
The Ayurvedic Institute, P.O. Box 23445
Albuquerque, New Mexico 87192-1445 (505) 291-9698

KITCHARI

Kitchari, a seasoned mixture of rice and mung dal, is basic to the Ayurvedic way of life. Both basmati rice and mung dal have the qualities of being sweet and cooling with a sweet aftertaste.

Together, they create a very balanced food that is an excellent protein combination and is tridoshic, which means that it is balancing for all three doshas: vata, pitta and kapha. This complete food is easy to digest and gives strength and vitality. It nourishes all the tissues of the body. Kitchari is the preferred food to use when fasting on a mono-fast or while going through cleansing programs such as pancakarma. Kitchari is excellent for detoxification and de-aging of the cells. The proportions are usually 2 parts rice to 1 part of dal, but both these and the spices can be varied according to need and constitution.

Yellow mung dal can be found at most oriental grocery stores. It is different from the green mung beans with which most people are familiar. This dal consists of hulled and split mung beans. Regular mung beans won't work as a substitute in this recipe because they are much more difficult to digest.

MUNG DAL KITCHARI

1 cup yellow mung dal
1 cup basmati rice
1 inch fresh ginger, peeled
1 tbs. shredded, unsweetened
  coconut
1 small handful fresh cilantro
  leaves
1 tbs. ghee
1 1/2 inch piece of cinnamon
  bark

1/2 cup of water
5 whole cardamom pods
5 whole cloves
10 black peppercorns
3 bay leaves
1/4 tsp. turmeric
1/4 tsp. salt
6 cups water

Wash mung dal and rice until water is clear. (Soaking the dal for a few hours helps with digestibility.) In a blender put the ginger, coconut, cilantro and 1/2 cup water and blend until liquefied. Heat a large sauce pan on medium heat and add ghee, cinnamon, cloves, cardamom, peppercorns and bay leaves. Stir for a moment until fragrant. Add the blended items to the spices, then the turmeric and salt. Stir until lightly browned. Stir in the mung dal and rice and mix very well. Pour in the 6 cups of water, cover, and bring to a boil. Let boil for 5 minutes, then turn heat down to very low and cook, lightly covered, until mung and rice are soft (25-30 minutes). Serves 4-5.

━━━━━━━━━━

Famous Vegetarians & Their Favorite Recipes
Lives & Lore from Buddha to the Beatles, by Rynn Berry
Pythagorean Books, G.P.O. Box 8174 JAF Station,
New York, NY 10116, USA

Berry's first book, *The Vegetarians,* is a collection of interviews with famous vegetarians. It created a small sensation when it came out. It was the subject of an essay in *Time* magazine and was selected for recommended reading by *Bon Appetit.* It also inspired a featured article in the Wednesday food section of *The New York Times* and was praised by *Library Journal,* as well as other journals throughout the U.S.

Famous Vegetarians is in the nature of a sequel. Having studied classical philology for several years in a post-graduate program in ancient studies at Columbia, Berry formed the habit of translating Greek and Latin authors for pleasure. This hobby stood him in good stead when it came to translating Leonardo da Vinci's recipes, which were written in Bartolomeo Platina's medieval Latin. It also enabled him to translate the relevant passages in Apicius, Plutarch, Porphyry and Pliny that are cited in *Famous Vegetarians.*

MATTAR PANEER WITH DEEP FRIED TOFU CUBES

1 lb. firm tofu	1 tbs. ginger, chopped fine
1 tsp. black mustard seed	1 tsp. garam masala
1 tsp. cumin seed	1 tsp. turmeric
4 cloves	2 green chili peppers, chopped
1 inch stick cinnamon	1 tsp. salt
1 medium with onion, chopped	1 tbs. fresh basil, chopped
	4 cups fresh, shelled peas
1 cup fresh tomatoes, peeled	1 tsp. coriander powder
2 cloves garlic, minced	

First press the tofu by placing it under a cutting board with a five pound weight atop it. Press for one half hour, then cut it into half-inch cubes. In a heavy skillet or fryer, deep fry the tofu cubes until they are golden. Remove with slotted spoon and drain on paper towels. While the tofu is being pressed, heat the hard spices—the mustard seeds, the cumin seeds, the cloves and the stick cinnamon until the mustard seed sputters and pops. Then add the chopped onions and fry until they turn transparent. As soon as the onions are ready, add the tomatoes and cook for about five minutes, then add garlic, ginger, garam masala, turmeric, green chilies, salt and basil. Cook for three more minutes and add the deep fried tofu cubes and fresh peas. Simmer over a medium flame until the peas have absorbed the cooking liquids. A few minutes before serving, stir in a teaspoonful of coriander powder. Serve with long-grain American rice or basmati rice.

Fields Of Greens
New Vegetarian Recipes from the Celebrated Greens Restaurant
by Annie Somerville, Bantam Books, 1540 Broadway New York , NY 10036. Anne Somerville is the executive chef at Greens of San Francisco.

"For beautifully prepared, superbly satisfying vegetarian fare, no restaurant compares with Greens. It is a major culinary landmark, elevating vegetables and grains to a new art form."
—from the *San Francisco Chronicle*

TAGLIARINI WITH ROASTED TOMATOES, GOLDEN ZUCCHINI, AND BASIL

The roasted tomatoes and their juice bring sweetness and intensity to this summer pasta. We like the flavor of Roma (plum) tomatoes and use them for this recipe. The tomatoes hold well, so you can roast them a day in advance, but don't try to hurry the roasting if you are running late.

Instead, substitute sun dried tomatoes. Garlic bread crumbs are a delicious addition.

1/2 pound golden zucchini or
  summer squash
1 pound roasted tomatoes
3 tbs. extra virgin olive oil
3 garlic cloves finely chopped
salt and pepper
1/2 tsp. hot pepper flakes

1/2 pound fresh tagliarini
2 tbs. pine nuts, toasted
15 to 20 fresh basil leaves,
  bundled and thinly sliced,
  about 1/3 cup
grated Parmesan cheese
1/2 cup bread crumbs

Set a large pot of water on the stove to boil. Cut the zucchini in half lengthwise and slice it diagonally into 1/2 inch thick pieces. (If you are using scalloped summer squash, such as sunburst or pattypan, cut it in half through the stem end and slice into 1/2 inch thick wedges.) Cut the roasted tomatoes in quarters or large pieces and reserve their juice for the sauce. Heat 2 tbs. of the olive oil in a large skillet and add the squash, garlic, 1/4 tsp. salt, and a few pinches of pepper. Sauté over medium high heat for about 2 to 3 minutes, just long enough to heat the squash through, then add the wine and cook for another minute, until the pan is nearly dry. Add the remaining olive oil, the tomatoes and their juice, 1/4 tsp. salt, and the hot pepper flakes. When the water is boiling, add 1 tsp. salt. Add the tagliarini and cook until just tender. Before you drain the pasta, add 1/4 cup of the cooking water to the sauté pan (this will make the sauce juicier).

Immediately drain the pasta, then add it to the tomatoes and squash along with the pine nuts and basil. Reduce the heat, toss well, and add salt and pepper to taste. Sprinkle with Parmesan and bread crumbs and serve immediately.

Roasted Tomatoes. Roma (plum) tomatoes roast particularly well because their flesh is dense and they are not very juicy. This recipe requires very little effort, and the full, intense flavor of the tomatoes is well worth the slow roasting time. They are a truly delicious addition to pasta, soups, stews, or cannellini beans; be sure to use every drop of their sweet juice. Since they hold well for up to a week, you may want to double the recipe and use the tomatoes in a variety of dishes.

1 pound Roma (plum) tomatoes
extra virgin olive oil

Preheat the oven to 250°F. Core the tomatoes and cut them in half crosswise. Squeeze them gently to drain their juice and remove the seeds. Place the tomatoes cut side down on a lightly oiled baking sheet. Roast for 2 hours, until the tomatoes are very shrunken. As they slowly roast, their flesh will shrink and the skink will shrivel, but they should not brown or burn. Use them immediately or refrigerate in a sealed container. Makes 1 cup. Line the baking sheet with parchment paper to keep the juice of the tomatoes from cooking onto the pan. We use this technique for roasting peppers as well; it makes cleaning the pan very easy.

━━━━━━━━

Food For Peace
Super Simple Vegetarian Cooking for Everyone
by Rambhoru Devi, Freedom Press, ISKCON—Center for Vedic Studies—Vrindavana U.P. 281124 India

CUSTARD SAMOSAS

Filling:
1/2 cup cornstarch or custard
powder
1/4 cup water
1 1/2 cups milk
3/4 cup sugar
1/2 cup tsp. vanilla essence
Mix corn starch and water,
stir in milk, sugar and

vanilla. Boil and stir until
thick. Remove from heat.
Spread on tray to cool.

Dough:
2 cups white flour
2 tsp. sugar
4 tbs. butter
1/2 cup cold water

Sift flour and sugar, rub in butter evenly, knead water into flour until a pliable dough forms. Divide dough into 12 balls. Lightly grease rolling surface. Roll each ball into a thin round. On lower half of round put 1 tbs. filling, leaving rim free. Rub a slight film of water around border. Fold top half of round over filling, matching up edges. Press along edges to seal. Do not squeeze filling as you go around. Starting at right corner of half moon, pinch and twist sealed edges in successive folds to form a fluted skirting. Each samosa must be well sealed not to break open during frying.

Heat deep fryer to moderate. Slip samosas into ghee. Fry until golden. Remove with a slotted spoon. Drain. Cool dip in carob Glaze. Carob glaze: 1/3 cup melted butter, 4 tbs. carob powder, 2 cups icing sugar, 1 1/2 tsp.. vanilla essence, 4-6 tbs. hot water. Melt butter. Remove from heat. Stir in carob, sugar and vanilla. Stir in water, until creamy. Yields 12 samosas.

Great Vegetarian Dishes
by Kurma dasa, The Bhaktivedanta Book Trust

VEGETARIAN SHEPHERD'S PIE

Those of you of Anglo-Saxon background, like myself, will perhaps be familiar with the non-vegetarian origins of the dish.

For base of pie:
1 1/4 cups (310 ml) brown lentils
2 litters / quarts water
1 tsp. (5 ml) yellow asafetida powder
1/4 tsp. (1 ml) freshly ground black pepper
1 cup (250 ml) celery, diced
home-made curd cheese (panir) from 8 cups (2 litters) milk and pressed for
1/2 hour
5 tbs. (100 ml) soy sauce
For potato topping:
6 large baking potatoes, peeled and cubed
2 tbs. (40 ml) butter
1/2 cup (125 ml) milk
1 tsp. (5 ml) salt
2 tbs. (40 ml) sour cream
3 tbs. (60 ml) chopped fresh parsley

Boil the brown lentils and water in a heavy 6 liter/quart saucepan. Reduce to a simmer and cook until they become soft. Strain through a colander. Put the lentils aside and retain the liquid for use as a soup stock at a later date

---

Higher Taste
A Guide to Gourmet Vegetarian Cooking and a Karma-Free Diet, based on the teachings of His Divine Grace A. C. Bhaktivedanta Swami Prabhupada, Founder-Acarya of The International Society for Krishna Consciousness. Published by the Bhaktivedanta Book Trust.

KOFTA BALLS IN TOMATO SAUCE

Sauce:

3 pounds tomatoes, blended (preferably Italian, plum type)	2 tsp. sweet basil
	2 tsp. salt
	1 tsp. turbinado sugar
1/4 cup olive oil	1/4 tsp. black pepper
2 tbs. butter	2 bay leaves
1/2 tsp. hing	1 pound spaghetti
1 medium carrot, cut in 8 pieces	

Heat oil and butter over medium heat. Add hing and fry for 30 seconds. Add carrot pieces and fry for 1 minute. Stir in the blended tomatoes and bring to a boil, then reduce the heat and simmer for 1 hour. Remove carrot pieces and bay leaves.

Kofta:	1/2 teaspoon hing
2 cups grated cauliflower	1 tsp. garam masala
2 cups grated cabbage	1 tsp. ground cumin
1 1/2 cups garbanzo bean flour	1/2 tsp. coriander powder
1 1/2 cups garbanzo bean flour	1/2 tsp. turmeric
1 1/2 tsp. salt	pinch of cayenne
	ghee or oil for deep frying

Heat ghee in a wok or 2 quart saucepan. Combine all of the ingredients in a bowl. Roll in 24 balls, 1 inch in diameter. Place as many balls in the ghee as possible, leaving enough room for them to float comfortably. Fry over medium heat for 10 minutes, until the kofta is a rich golden brown. Drain in colander. Place the kofta in the tomato sauce

5 minutes before serving. If after sitting the kofta soaks up most of the sauce, add a little water to produce more liquid. You can also serve kofta and sauce over spaghetti. Serves 4

━━━━━━━━

Kathy Cooks, by Kathy Hoshijo
ISBN 0-671-67805-1, A Fireside Book (Simon and Schuster) 1986

Following Japanese tradition, my mother used to serve miso soup for breakfast sometimes. It's a fairly quick breakfast to make the night before and simply heat up in the morning. (It's good cold on hot summer days.)

The Amazing Power of Miso
In the very interesting book *Diet for the Atomic Age—How to Protect Yourself from Low-Level Radiation*, Sara Shannon, presenting the incredible healing power of miso, recalls what happened in 1945 in the Saint Francis clinic in Japan, not far from the place hit by the A-bomb.

"I had fed my workers," explained Dr. Azizuki, "brown rice and miso soup for some time before the bombing. None of them suffered from atomic radiation. I believe this is because they had eaten miso soup. It was thanks to this method that all of us could work away for people day after day, overcoming fatigue or symptoms of atomic disease, and survived the disaster free from severe symptoms of radioactivity."

In 1981, the National Cancer Center of Japan, after thirteen years of research, confirmed the radioprotective power of miso.

Miso contains dipicolinic acid which grabs onto heavy metals (radioactive strontium being one) and discharges them from the body. Miso can also help to neutralize the effects of air pollution.

MISO SOUP

12 cups water
1 foot strip of kombu seaweed
1/2 cup slivered carrots

3 cups mild-flavored Chinese
 green (such as Chinese
 cabbage) cut in 1" pieces

2 cups watercress or Chinese mustard greens cut in 1" chunks	**1 cup sliced, fresh mushrooms** **1 1/2 cups dark miso** **1 block tofu, cubed**

Bring first 2 ingredients to a boil. (Use whole 1 foot strip of kombu seaweed if you want to remove it from the soup before serving; otherwise, cut it into fine julienne strips.) Then begin adding other ingredients to the water in the order listed. If not using ingredients specified in this recipe, just remember to add the hardest vegetables first since they will take longer to cook, and then end with the vegetables that cook very quickly. If you add each vegetable just after it's cut, the timing works out perfectly. To add miso, place miso inside of a fairly fine-screened strainer. Immerse bottom part of strainer into boiling water and mash miso through the screen into the water with the back of a large spoon. This makes a smoother soup. Add cubes of tofu and cook long enough to warm.

Serve with a scoop of brown rice or brown rice crackers. Makes six 2 cup servings.

―――――――――――

Lord Krishna's Cuisine:The Art of Indian Vegetarian Cooking
by Yamuna Devi, Bala Books - E. P. Dutton

Yamuna's first experience with Indian vegetarian cooking came in New York, in 1966. She met Bhaktivedanta Swami Prabhupada. "Besides being a Sanskrit scholar, teacher, and saintly person," she recalls, "he was an excellent cook."

Yamuna traveled with him across India and learned to cook from him and other experts. Traveling to many obscure and exotic places, she studied recipes and techniques that have been employed in ancient temples for centuries. The value of her experience is clear. A few years back, in 1987, in a radical break from its meat-centered tradition, the esteemed members of the International Association of Cooking Professionals (IACP) conferred upon Yamuna their organization's most prestigious award, the "IACP Cookbook of the Year" for her 800-page work, *Lord Krishna's Cuisine.* In 1988, the same book was honored with the "Benjamin Franklin Award" for cookbooks.

In 1992, her second book, *Yamuna's Table* (E.P. Dutton), which focused on quick and light vegetarian cuisine, won the James Beard Award for the "Best International Cookbook."

"There is a spiritual dimension to vegetarianism that sees the world as a living planet in which all species are interdependent. People are beginning to understand that proper vegetarian eating is better for their health. But when I explain the callousness of the meat industry and what it's doing to our environment, it penetrates to their deepest sense of conscience. What I call spiritual vegetarianism can be one of the most positive approaches to avoid ecological disaster."

OUKI SHORBA
ZUCCHINI CUBES IN LIGHT TOMATO BROTH

In India, wrote Yamuna, this dish would be made with young bottle gourd (louki) or round gourd (tinda). If you live near a good Indian green grocery, by all means try both kinds. Zucchini should be young and seedless. Basil complements any summer-type squash. Native to India, sweet basil is found profusely in one form or another throughout the country. It is not, however, commonly used in cooking. Two of the three most popular varieties—the purple-leafed Krishna Tulsi (Ocimum Sanctum) and the green-leafed Rama Tulsi (Ocimum albuin) are never used in cooking. They are sacred plants, kept for the worship of Lord Krishna, and are cared for with reverence. The shiny, pale green-leafed variety of camphor basil (Ocimum kilimandscharicum) is used in cooking. It is always used fresh; in the Himalayan foothills, cooks purchase it daily, along with coriander, mint or curry leaves and a handful of green chilies and ginger root. In America, it is encouraging to see fresh herbs as these are becoming more common in supermarkets and specialty green groceries. They are also easy to grow in a kitchen window sill garden and flourish in hydroponic containers.

This dish, laced with both fresh sweet basil and coriander, is an example of simple New Indian cooking at its best. Serve it with a grain pilaf and flatbreads for a light lunch. Preparation time (after assembling ingredients): 10 minutes. Cooking time: 15 minutes. Serves: 4 or 5

1/2 tbs. (7 ml) scraped,
minced fresh ginger root
2 hot green chilies, seeded and
minced (or as desired)
2 tbs. (30 ml) tomato paste
1 1/4 tsps (6 ml) crushed dry-
roasted cumin seeds
1 tsp. (5 ml) garam masala
1/8 tsp. (0.5 ml) paprika or
cayenne pepper
1/2-1 tsp. (2-5 ml) salt

3/4 cup (180 ml) water
3/4 cup (180 ml) half and half
or light cream
3 tbs. (45 ml) ghee or unsalted
butter
6-7 small zucchini (about 1
pound/455 gm), trimmed
and cut into 1/2 inch (1.5
cm) cubes
1/2 tbs. 922 ml) each chopped
fresh sweet basil and
coriander.

Combine the ginger, chilies, tomato paste, cumin, garam masala, paprika or cayenne and salt in a mixing bowl. Slowly stir in 1/2 cup (120 ml) of the water, blend.

Yamuna gave us a full detailed description of ghee, an important ingredient of the Indian kitchen.

How To Make Ghee

I have made hundreds of pots of ghee in the last thirty years, and I always enjoy doing it. Preparing ghee is so easy and saves so much money that I rarely buy ghee. Like other fine-quality oils in my kitchen, most of my batches of ghee are flavor-infused with herbs or spices. My current favorite is made with cloves, cinnamon, and fresh curry leaves. I often make extra to bottle as gifts. Of course, the quality of the ghee rests on the quality of the butter, so use the best available. You can get organic unsalted butter in some large natural-food stores, and you can always try to find a local organic dairy that has it. To infuse ghee with flavor, for every pound of ghee you make add one, two, or even three of the following seasonings.

3-4 sprigs of fresh curry
leaves
7-8 whole cloves
13-inch cinnamon stick
2-3 tsps of whole peppercorns
1 1-inch piece of sliced ginger

1 large dried chili, such as
chilpote, New Mexico, or
Ancho.
1 tbs. of toasted cumin or
coriander seeds
4-6 generous sprigs of mint or
cilantro

Place all of the butter in a heavy-bottomed saucepan, with the surface of the butter at least 2 inches below the rim of the pan. Melt the butter over moderate heat and bring to a gentle boil until the butter is covered with foam.

Reduce the heat to very low, and simmer the butter uncovered, stirring occasionally. Cook until the casein solids have settled to the bottom of the pan and turned from white to rich brown. A thin transparent crust should appear on the surface of the clear, golden, near-motionless ghee. (Toward the end of cooking, watch closely to prevent burning.)

With a skimmer remove the crust and set it aside to use in rice, legumes, or vegetables. With a ladle remove all but the bottom inch of clear ghee and pour it into a sealable container through a coffee filter or a fine sieve lined with a paper towel. Then pour the rest of the ghee from the pot, stopping just short of the brown solids. When the ghee has cooled to room temperature, seal the container well. The ghee will keep for a few months at cool to moderate room temperature. When the weather is warm, keep the ghee in the refrigerator.

Removing the casein from butter has the advantage of holding down cholesterol. Pure ghee contains no lactose or oxidized cholesterol. Though you are best off checking with your doctor, many lactose-intolerant people find little or no difficulty digesting ghee. Since ghee has no casein, it is similar to many nut or vegetable oils.

Ghee contains beta carotene and vitamins A, D, E, and K. Betacarotene and vitamin E are both valuable antioxidants that help fight off disease and injury. Besides ghee, no edible fat except fish oil (if you consider that edible) contains vitamin A, which helps maintain good vision and keeps the outer lining of the eyeballs moist. Ghee contains four to five percent linoleic acid, which helps the body properly grow and develop. Linoleic acid is an essential fatty acid often lacking in a vegetarian diet.

Modern research backs up the kitchen granny wisdom that mixing herbs and spices with ghee makes the herbs and spices more useful and beneficial. One or two daily teaspoons of ghee improves digestion, helps assimilation and nourishes the brain.

The only brand of ready-made ghee I buy is organic. It comes from Purity Farms, Inc., 14635 Westercreek Road, Sedalia, CO 80135, phone (303) 647-2368. It is available at many large natural food and grocery stores.

Yamuna Devi is an award-winning author and regular contributor to *The Washington Post*, *Vegetarian Times* and *Back to Godhead*.

The New McDougall Cookbook
by Mary McDougall (Dutton Publishers, 1993)

SEITAN BOURGUIGNON

3 medium onions, sliced
1/2 pound mushrooms, sliced
1/2 cup water   2 cups cubed seitan
1 cup nonalcoholic red wine
1 1/2 cups vegetable broth (or liquid from making seitan)
1/3 cup soy sauce

1/4 tsp. dried marjoram
1/4 tsp. dried thyme
1/8 tsp. freshly ground black pepper
2 1/2 tbs. cornstarch, mixed with 1/4 cup water

Place the onion and mushrooms in a large pot with the water. Sauté for about 15 minutes, or until tender. Add the remaining ingredients, except the cornstarch mixture. Cover and cook over medium-low heat for about 45 minutes. Add the cornstarch mixture. Cook, stirring, until thickened.

Serves 6 to 8. Preparation time: 15 minutes (need prepared seitan). Cooking time: 1 hour. Serve over rice, pasta, potatoes, or bread.

"Most people of Western societies are fat and sick because they eat like the kings and queens of old—every day. Their meals are filled with meat, poultry, fish, eggs, and dairy products, topped off by cookies and cakes, and washed down with glasses of milk. All that feasting has undeniable adverse consequences. Fortunately, the human body is a miracle, blessed with an astounding ability to heal itself when cared for properly. Obesity, high blood pressure, adult diabetes, arthritis, intestinal distress, and heart disease are only a few of the problems solved by proper eating. The foods that result in health and healing are low-fat, pure-vegetarian. The right diet is based around starchy vegetable foods with the addition of fruits and vegetables delightfully seasoned."
—John McDougall, M.D.

The Now And Zen Epicure
Gourmet Cuisine for the Enlightened Palate
by Miyoko Nishimoto, Book Publishing Company, Summertown, Tennessee.

Miyoko is also managing a successful restaurant in San Francisco, Now & Zen, 1826 Buchanan Street, tel:(415) 922-9696   fax: (415) 922-1343.

"If nouvelle cuisine has a vegetarian counterpart, the Now and Zen recipes are definitely it."
—*San Francisco Examiner*

This book is a landmark for vegetarian cooking, inspired by the best of French and Japanese culinary traditions. A guide for preparing delicious and elegant cuisine, featured are gourmet dishes for the most discriminating palate.

WHOLE CABBAGE WITH HEARTY TEMPEH STUFFING

This will warm you on a cold winter day. It's also a fun dish to serve because a beautifully sauced head of cabbage is cut open at the table to reveal a "meaty" filling. The tomato sauce is also fat-free, although rich and tasty.

1 medium head cabbage
 (approx. 2 lb.)
12 oz. tempeh, minced or
 crumbled
2 tbs. cider vinegar
2 tsps honey
3 tbs. soy sauce
1 tbs. sake (optional)
1/4 tsp. dry mustard or 1 tsp.
 prepared mustard
2 tbs. oil

1 medium onion minced
1 cup cooked brown rice
3-4 cloves garlic, minced
1/2 tsp. thyme
1/4 tsp. sage
3 tbs. tomato paste
2 oz. walnuts, ground
1 tbs. miso
freshly ground pepper
2 additional tbs. soy sauce
 (optional)

Tomato Sauce:
1 lb. very ripe tomatoes (may
   substitute canned)
1 1/4 cups water from boiling
   cabbage
3/4 cup red wine

2 tbs. soy sauce
2 tbs. mirin
1/2 tbs. honey
1/2 tbs. miso

To core the cabbage, cut out a small cone at the core with a sharp knife. Fill a large pot that will hold the entire head of cabbage half full with water. Bring it to a boil and add the cored cabbage.

After the water reboils, simmer the cabbage for about ten minutes. With two forks, start removing the leaves of the cabbage, being careful not to tear them too badly—some tearing is inevitable. They should come off easily. Remove 14 to 16 leaves and set them aside to drain in a colander.

Pierce the remaining cabbage (still cooking in water), and if it seems raw or undercooked, boil a few more minutes. If it is tender, remove it and set aside to cool. The cabbage should be tender but still slightly crisp—not mushy. When cool enough to handle, shred or chop it finely. Reserve 1 1/4 cups of the cooking water for later.

Mix the tempeh with the vinegar, honey, soy sauce, sake, and mustard, and sauté it in the oil lightly browned. Add the minced onion and continue to sauté until tender about 10 minutes. Add the remaining ingredients including the chopped cabbage, but not the leaves. Season to taste with plenty of freshly ground pepper and the additional two tablespoons of soy sauce, if necessary.

Grease a glass or earthenware round casserole dish and line it with 6 of the outer leaves, allowing the edges to extend beyond the rim of the dish so they can be folded over the top later. Trim the hard rib of the leaves if necessary to make them more pliable. Pack half the tempeh filling into this, then neatly arrange about 4 leaves on top, again cutting away the rib, if desired. Pack the rest of the tempeh mixture in tightly and arrange the remaining leaves over the top ones. Weigh down with a heavy plate or lid and cover everything with aluminum foil. Bake at 375 degrees for 1 1/4 hours.

While the cabbage bakes, mix all the ingredients for the sauce and simmer gently, covered, for 30 to 40 minutes. Puree in a blender or food processor, then return to the sauce pan and simmer for another 10 minutes, or until thick enough to coat the back of a wooden spoon (boil down if necessary).

To serve, invert the cabbage onto a platter. You should have a shining, glimmering head of cabbage that will look delicious. Pour several tablespoons of the sauce on top, letting it dribble down like frosting on a cake. Cut the cabbage in wedges like a pie and pass the remaining sauce around for individual servings. Per serving: Calories: 324, Protein: 15 gm., Carbohydrates: 31 gm.

Simple Food For The Good Life
by Helen Nearing. Good Life Center, Harborside, Maine 04642 USA

"I had the good sense, or good luck, to be born to vegetarian parents and I can't imagine eating any other way. With fruits and nuts and vegetables everywhere available, why eat brother animals? My husband, Scott, for 70 years a convinced vegetarian, lived to the honorable age of 100. Now (March '95) at 91, I am still active in house and garden, travel the world over, and just finished my sixth book, and may get to another. Long live the vegetarian way!"

MIRACLE MUSH

2 apples, unpeeled	**1 beet**
1 carrot	**1/4 cup grated nuts**

Grate apples, carrot and beet together. Sprinkle with nuts. If too dry, moisten with apple or orange juice.

Simply Vegan, Quick Vegetarian Meals, by Debra Wasserman
The Vegetarian Resource Group, Box 1463, Baltimore, MD 21203

Easy vegan recipes, a complete vegan nutrition section, and a list of where to mail-order vegan food, clothing, cosmetics, and household products. Vegan menus and meal plans.

GARBANZO BEAN BURGERS

2 cups pre-cooked garbanzo   1/4 small onion, minced
  beans (chickpeas)   1/4 cup whole wheat flour
1 stalk celery, finely chopped   salt and pepper to taste
1 carrot, finely chopped   2 tsp. oil

Mash the garbanzo beans in a large bowl. Add the remaining ingredients, except the oil. Mix well. Form 6 flat patties. Fry in oiled pan over medium-high heat until burgers are golden brown on each side. Serve on whole wheat buns with lettuce and tomato, or alone with a mushroom gravy, ketchup, or barbecue sauce.

Soul Vegetarian Cookbook

From the Kitchens of Soul Vegetarian, published by Communicators Press, P.O. Box 26063, Washington, D.C. 20001   (202) 726-8618   fax (202) 291-9149.

This cookbook is from the African Hebrew Israelite Community of Jerusalem. They believe that what is called Eden in the Old Testament was actually in Africa. Israelites lived in Eden and were vegetarian in accordance with Scripture. They also believe that a vegetarian diet coincides with the highest form of spirituality. After the Romans took control of Jerusalem, 70 A.D., the Israelites dispersed throughout the world. Today, the African Hebrew Israelite Community is headquartered in Israel and numbers about 2,000 members worldwide. The community operates vegan restaurants in Tel Aviv, Washington D.C., Atlanta (879 A Ralph Abernathy Blvd, SW, GA 30310) and Chicago (205 E. 75th Street, IL 60619).

DOWN-SOUTH BARBECUE TWISTS

2 lb. seitan dough from packaged seitan mix or Homemade
  Seitan (a chewy, meat-like, high protein food made from boiled
  or baked wheat gluten—available in dry mixes, prepared
  chilled in the deli section and prepared frozen).

1/4 cup nutritional yeast (A dietary supplement and condiment that has a distinct but pleasant aroma. Its taste varies from nutty to cheesy. It can be added to soups and casseroles or sprinkled on toast, popcorn or spaghetti.)

1/3 cup natural-style smooth peanut butter or tahini
1 tbs. paprika
1 tbs. garlic powder
1 onion, minced
1/4 cup warmed canola oil
1/2 cup Barbecue Sauce

In large bowl, pull and stretch seitan dough; mix in nutritional yeast, peanut butter, paprika and garlic powder. When ingredients are incorporated and dough is elastic and smooth, let rest a few minutes.

Meanwhile, sauté onion over medium heat in oil until transparent, about 5 minutes. While onion-oil mixture is still warm, mix with seitan dough by pulling and stretching. Pull and stretch until texture is stringy but dough doesn't tear, about 5 minutes. Preheat oven to 350 degrees. Cut gluten into 12 pieces. Stretch and twist pieces around 12 bamboo skewers that have been soaked into water. Place twists on lightly oiled baking sheet. Bake 30 minutes; brush twists with Barbecue Sauce and bake 10 minutes longer. Makes 12 twists.

Per serving: 356 cal; 43 g prot; 6 g fat; 34 g carb; 0 chol; 152 mg sod; 5 g fiber

Barbecue Sauce

2 tbs. margarine or canola oil, the market name for rapeseed oil. (It is mild flavored and lower in saturated fat than any other oil.)
3 tbs. molasses
1 tbs. apple cider vinegar
1 cup water
1 bay leaf

12-oz. can tomato paste
4 tbs. honey or brown sugar
2 tbs. garlic powder
1/8 cup tamari, a naturally brewed soy sauce that contains no sugar—available wheat-free
salt to taste

Place all ingredients in medium saucepan. Simmer over low heat 20 minutes. Makes 2 cups. Per Tablespoon: 33 cal; 1 g prot; 1 g fat; 7 g carb; 0 chol; 103 mg sod; 1 g fiber.

Homemade Seitan　　　　　**2 lb. whole wheat flour**
　　　　　　　　　　　　　1 quart water

In large bowl, mix flour and water thoroughly (consistency should be medium to firm). Let dough rest at least 45 minutes. Put dough in colander. While running cold water, continually squeeze dough to wash out starch from mixture. Dough should remain intact in one piece during squeezing. Keep rinsing and squeezing until all graininess is gone and water runs clear, 10 to 15 minutes. Cover seitan with water until ready to use. Makes 12 servings. Per serving: 284 cal; 40 g prot; 2 g fat; 26 g carb; 0 chol; 38 mg sod; 4 g fiber.

Soups For All Seasons
Bountiful Vegetarian Soups, by Nava Atlas
Amberwood Press, 65 Prospect Street, New Paltz, NY 12561-1143

SWEET POTATO SOUP

2 tbs. margarine　　　　　　**2 bay eaves**
2 medium onions　　　　　　　**1/4 tsp. dried thyme**
2 medium carrots, diced　　　**1/4 tsp. ground nutmeg**
1 large celery stalk, diced　　**1 cup low fat milk or soy milk,**
handful of celery leaves　　　　　**or as needed**
6 cups diced (1/2 inch) sweet　**salt and freshly ground**
　potatoes　　　　　　　　　　　**pepper to taste**

Heat the margarine in a large soup pot. Add the onions, carrots, and celery and sauté over low heat until the onions are golden. Add the celery leaves and sweet potato dice. Add just enough water to cover all but about 1 inch of the vegetables. Bring to a boil, then stir in the bay leaves and seasonings. Simmer over moderate heat until the sweet potatoes and vegetables are tender, about 20 minutes.　With a slotted spoon, remove about half of the solid ingredients and transfer to a food processor along with about 1/2 cup of the cooking liquid. Process until smoothly pureed, then stir back into the soup pot. Add the milk or soymilk as needed to achieve a slightly consistency. Season to taste with salt and pepper. Simmer over very low heat for another 10 to 15 minutes.

━━━━━━━━

Vegetarian Food For All
by Annabel Perkins
New World Library, 14 Pamaron Way, Novato California 94949.
(415) 884-2100 fax (415) 884-2199

From the famous vegetarian restaurant Food for All, this cookbook offers cooks a collection of tasty international recipes to expand their vegetarian repertoire. Chef Annabel Perkins collected the most mouth-watering results of those culinary experiments.

EGGPLANT WALNUT DIP

1 large eggplant	**pinch cayenne pepper, or a**
1/2 c walnuts	**dash of hot pepper sauce**
2 tbs. olive oil	**parsley or watercress to**
salt and pepper to taste	**garnish.**
1 tsp. paprika	

Prick eggplant, wrap in foil. Bake whole for about 40 minutes at 350 F until tender. Put walnuts in the oven and bake for 5 minutes with eggplant, then chop finely or grind. When the eggplant is done, cut in half and scoop out the flesh. Place the flesh in a blender with oil, salt, pepper, paprika, and cayenne and combine. When smooth, turn into a bowl, mix with walnuts, garnish and serve. Serves 4-6

━━━━━━━━

The Vegetarian Lunch Basket, by Linda Haynes
New World Library, Pamaron Way, Novato CA 94990.
225 easy, nutritious recipes for the quality-conscious family on the go.

"The Vegetarian Lunch Basket is lots of fun and full of terrific lunch ideas. If you are stuck in a rut of packing peanut butter sand-

wiches every day, this book will pull you out of it—permanently! This is family food—hearty and unpretentious."
—*Vegetarian Times*

SQUASH CHEESE SOUP

3 tbs. butter (or margarine)
3 tbs. whole wheat flour
2 cups milk (or vegetable stock)
1 cup grated sharp cheddar

cheese
2 cups cooked winter squash, mashed
salt and pepper to taste

In a saucepan, melt butter and whisk in flour. Slowly add milk or broth while stirring and simmer until thickened. Stir in cheese, squash, and seasonings. Simmer 5 minutes more.

Vegetarian Times Complete Cookbook
by the Editors of *Vegetarian Times* (MacMillan, 1995).
Order Toll Free: 800-358-6327

This 500+ page book includes mouth-watering recipes and cutting-edge nutrition information for everyone, from those seeking to cut meat out of their diets to long-time vegans. Here is a sampling of what you will find:
• More than 600 appetizer, entrees and dessert recipes
• An easy-to-understand guide to vegetarian health and nutrition
• A glossary of vegetarian ingredients
• Low-fat cooking techniques
• How to plan delicious vegetarian menus
• Ethical reasons for not eating meat

Vegetarian Times is a monthly magazine selling hundreds of thousands of copies. Editorial Offices: P.O. Box 570, Oak Park, IL 60303, (708) 848-8100, fax (708) 848-2031   E-mail:74651.215@compuserve.com (74651.215 within Compu-Serve). Subscription orders and information 800-435-9610; from outside the U.S. call (815) 734-5824

"Earlier this year, when the U.S. Department of Agriculture and Department of Health and Human Services released their new dietary guidelines, my phone rang off the hook because the guidelines had, for the first time, used the V-word (vegetarian). Finally, a vegetarian diet had the sanction of the U.S. government! What a relief to the more than 12 million vegetarians who have been living healthy lives all along, thank you, and most of whom didn't need to be told by the government that their diet is OK. They knew it all along. Most of the calls came from reporters and others not familiar with a vegetarian diet, asking if I was thrilled to see this kind of progress. Thrilled? Progress? The most pertinent question was this: 'Why do you think the U.S. government decided to speak to the healthfulness of vegetarian diets now?' I thought a minute. Then I got angry.

'Because the scientific research and the medical evidence that a vegetarian diet is more healthful than one that includes meat is absolutely overwhelming and I think that even bureaucrats can no longer ignore it. To do so would be gross negligence,' I blurted out."

The one helpful statement in the guidelines—'Enjoy meals that have rice, pasta , potatoes or bread at the center of the plate, accompanied by vegetables and fruit, and lean and low-fat foods from the other groups'—didn't get picked up in the popular press and very few of us will ever see that advice in print.

"Luise Light, Ed.D., who served on the first guidelines committee back in 1980 and who is currently director of the Institute for Science in Society in Kensington, Md., suggests a national hotline, similar to the National Cancer Hotline, to help show people how to shop for, prepare and eat a more healthful diet. Better yet would be community-based hotlines staffed by knowledgeable pratictioners who can give useful advice to such common questions as, 'What about protein?' and 'What can I serve for breakfast besides bacon and eggs?'"

"Light throws out a challenge: 'Why can't your magazine be the catalyst for such change?' We can and we will. We'll need all of your support and your ideas. Write to me. Let's come up with a plan to take positive action to get the word out in ways that aren't being done right now. This is the right time and the right place to start."

—printed in *Vegetarian Times*, March 1996
by Toni Agpar, Editorial Director

Tofu Pumpkin Pie

This tasty version of a classic Thanksgiving dessert is egg- and dairy-free. Candied ginger adds a festive touch.

Crust:
2 cups all-purpose flour
1/2 cup (1 stick) margarine or
  butter
1 tsp. salt
3 to 4 tbs. cold water

Combine the flour, margarine or butter, and salt in a food processor using the standard cutting blade. Process for 30 seconds using a standard cutting blade. Add the water through the feed tube and process the dough to form a ball. (Or, by hand, stir together the flour and salt in a bowl. Cut in the margarine or butter, and distribute evenly using a fork or your fingers. Add the water, stirring to form a ball.) Wrap the dough in plastic wrap or wax paper and chill at least 30 minutes. Then roll out the dough with a rolling pin and place it in a 10-inch tart pan or a deep-dish pie pan. Set aside.

Filling:
1 pound firm tofu
one 16-ounce can pureed
  pumpkin
1 tsp. ground cinnamon
1/4 tsp. ground nutmeg
1/2 tsp. salt
1 tsp. vanilla extract
3/4 cup light brown sugar
1/4 tsp. ground cloves
1/3 cup safflower oil
5 Tbs. candied ginger,
  chopped (or 1 tsp. ground
  ginger)

Preheat the oven to 350°F. Combine all the filling ingredients except the candied ginger in a food processor or blender. (If using ground ginger, add it at this time.) Process until smooth, about 3 minutes. Add 3 Tbs. candied ginger, and process 30 seconds more. Pour the filling into the crust and bake 1 hour. Let cool. Place the remaining 2 Tbs. candied ginger in the food processor or blender and process until coarsely ground. Sprinkle over the pie. Serve warm or chilled.

Per Serving: 203 cal, 6 g Protein, 13 g Fat, 38 g Carb, 440 mg Sod, 1 g Fiber, 0 mg Chol.

"Having been introduced to vegetarianism in the 1960's in San Francisco, and now working full-time in the field as a vegetarian food editor, my commitment to the vegetarian life style grows stronger daily. How could it not? Vegetarianism helps the planet environmentally; lessens animal suffering; allows me to be as healthy as possible; and I get to eat all my favorite ethnic foods. And as long as I eat sensibly, I can eat whatever I want whenever I want without having to be overly concerned with counting calories or fat. So why isn't everyone vegetarian?"

—Karen Cope Straus, Food Editor of
Vegetarian Times

Thank You

for the time and attention that you have already dedicated to our project. This simple series of useful recipes and quotes can help rid the world of bad habits and allow you to personally enter a victorious phase in your life. Follow the good examples of those that have already applied this knowledge to great success. Reading is not enough. Now go back to your kitchen and—with a clearer conscience and consciousness—create a fresh, peaceful, loving environment. Cook, eat and feed naturally your precious body. You can have many houses and many cars but the body you live in is the only one this life....

This book is a combined effort of many intelligent and successful people; they are all your good friends. Believe that God gave the gift of life to all sentient beings—human and animal. Each one of the billions of animals killed every year is an individual, fully capable of feeling deeply the boredom, stress, pain, thirst, fear and panic imposed on him or her. Animals experience pleasure and pain in much the same way as we humans. They too have faces and families. With this compassionate mood, enjoy a happy and healthy life—and share this knowledge with all the people you love. Be honest and sincere, promise to God, yourself and others: "NO MORE KILLING."

If you enjoyed this book we feel sure you will also enjoy our other titles listed at the back. Take a look now!

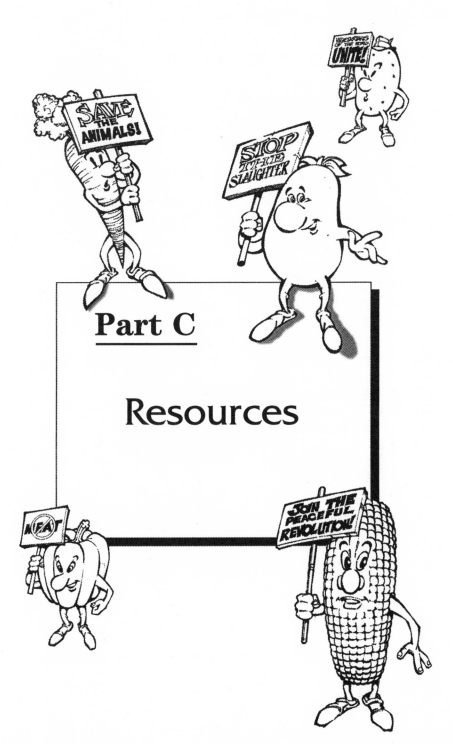

Part C

Resources

VEGETARIANS INTERNATIONAL
Feeding People With Love Worldwide

Vegetarians International
President
Giorgio Cerquetti

NORTH AMERICA
Vegetarians International
Alister Taylor
P.O. Box 45
Badger, California 93603
Tel. 209 337-2200
Fax 209 337-2354

Vegetarians International
Rynn Berry
159 Eastern Parkway Suite 2h
Brooklyn, New York 11238
Tel. 718-622-8002

SOUTH AMERICA
Vegetarians International
Raphael Lopez Seco
General Pinto 1586
San Fernando
Buenos Aires, ARGENTINA

EUROPE
Vegetarians International
Giulia Amici
Via Bonazza 11
Tavarnelle V.P.
50028 Firenze, ITALY
Tel. 055-8077701

Vegetarians International
Nicole Barthelmy
Via Catalani 31
Roma, ITALY
Tel. 06-86-20-9531

ASIA
Vegetarians International
Paola Mosconi
c/o Jhanava Devi
Sri Krishna Mission School
Village Sonatala
PO Bamuthin
Tripura (W) 799211
INDIA
Tel. 0091-381-223891

Alphabetical Listing of Recipe Sources

Recipes from People

1 Minestrone Soup: Giulia Amici
2 Food for the Sufis — Three Bean Curry: Muhaiyaddeen Bawa
3 Watercress Salad Sandwich: Annie Besant
4 Cauliflower Pakoras: Bhaktivedanta Swami
5 Lentil Soup: Edward Espe Brown
6 Mung Beans and Rice: Lord Buddha
7 Nut Loaf: Peter Burwash
8 Bunchi Moong Dal Kichari: Caitanya Mahaprabhu
9 Vegetarian Chicken Salad: Greg Caton
10 Pasta Arame with Oyster Mushrooms: Lee Chamberlin
11 Coconut Burfi: Deen B. Chandora
12 Sunflower Seed Cheese: Terry Cole-Whittaker
13 Mango Dessert: Michael Cremo
14 Spicy Sauteed Tofu: Alfred Ford
15 Basic Vegan Curry Casserole: Michael Fox
16 Franciscan Chickpeas: Saint Francis of Assisi
17 Eggplant Spread: Phil Gallelli
18 Chapatis (whole wheat tortillas): Mahatma Gandhi
19 Baghare Baingam (Stuffed Eggplant): Maneka Gandhi
20 Seitan Stir Fries: Boy George
21 Eggplant Casserole: Arthur Goldberg
22 Mixed Salad: Dick Gregory
23 Dark Horse Lentil Soup: George Harrison
24 Astro Burger: James Higgins
25 Quince Jelly: John Hogue
26 Essene Sprouted Bread: Jesus Christ
27 Asparagus on Toast with Soy Cream Sauce: John Harvey Kellogg
28 Kasturi Sandesh (Pistachio Milk Sweet with Rose Water): Shri Krishna
29 Southern Style Spicy Kale with Vegan Cornbread: Rowena Pattee Kryder
30 Sweet and Pungent Vegetable Curry: k. d. lang
31 Chili Con Tofu: Frances Moore Lappe
32 Baked Cinnamon Apple Delight: Joy Irene Lasseter

Recipes from Groups

Recipes from Restaurants

16 Northeast African Millet Patties — Washington DC: Soul Vegetarian Cafe

Recipes from Books

1 Mung Dal Kitchari: *Ayurvedic Cooking for Self Healing* by Usha Lad & Vasant Lad
2 Mattar Paneer with Deep Fried Tofu Cubes: *Famous Vegetarians* by Rynn Berry
3 Tagliarini with Roasted Tomatoes, Golden Zucchini and Basil: *Fields of Greens* by Annie Sommerville
4 Custard Samosa: *Food for Peace* by Rambhoru Devi
5 Vegetarian Shepherd's Pie: *Great Vegetarian Dishes* by Kurma
6 Kofta Balls in Tomato Sauce: *Higher Taste* by ISKCON
7 Miso Soup: *Kathy Cooks* by Kathy Hoshijo
8 Ouki Shorba (Zucchini Cubes in Light Tomato Broth) and How to Make Ghee (clarified butter): *Lord Krishna's Cuisine* by Yamuna Devi
9 Seitan Bourguinon: *New McDougall Cookbook*
10 Whole Cabbage with Hearty Tempeh Stuffing and Tomato Sauce: *Now and Zen Epicure*
11 Miracle Mush: *Simple Food for the Good Life*
12 Garbanzo Bean Burgers: *Simply Vegan, Quick Vegetarian Meals*
13 Down-South Barbecue Twists and Barbecue Sauce: *Soul Vegetarian Cookbook*
14 Sweet Potato Soup: *Soups for All Seasons*
15 Eggplant Walnut Dip: *Vegetarian Food for All*
16 Squash Cheese Soup: *Vegetarian Lunch Basket*
17 Tofu Pumpkin Pie: *Vegetarian Times Complete Cookbook*

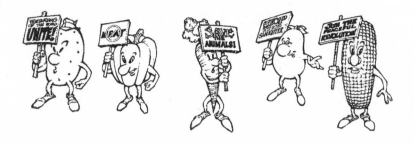

About the Author

Giorgio Cerquetti, Ph.D., author and yoga practitioner, was born in Italy in 1946 and has been a vegetarian since the age of sixteen. He has written books and numerous articles for major magazines and newspapers, and is a recognized television and radio personality in Italy, where he has been instrumental in introducing exciting new concepts for better living. Between 1968 and 1991 he lived part time in India, where he studied yoga, Vedic philosophy and the spiritual aspects of vegetarianism.

In 1991 Giorgio started to spend more time in the U.S.A. and with Alister Taylor he founded Vegetarians International. As president of Vegetarians International, a non-profit organization, he actively promotes vegetarianism, and is involved with food distribution to the needy worldwide. He travels between America and Europe giving lectures on vegetarianism, psychosomatic healing and meditation.

All profits from this book will be given to promote vegetarianism and free food distribution to the needy worldwide.

Diet For Transcendence

Vegetarianism and the World Religions

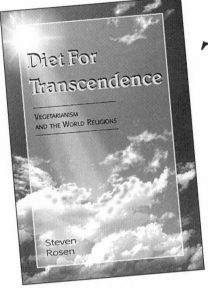

by Steven Rosen

$11.95 ISBN #1-887089-05-5
6"x 9", paper 156 pgs.

"Steven Rosen takes us on a fascinating journey back in time to explore the essential and often misunderstood roots of the world's major religious traditions, to discover how vegetarianism was a cherished part of their philosophy and practice."

Nathaniel Altman,
Author, *Eating for Life*

Following the Path of Kindness

This is reinforcement and inspiration for the 86% of the American population that is making a conscious effort to improve their diets by consuming more fruits and vegetables. Following an introductory overview of the physiological, environmental and economic reasons for adopting a vegetarian diet, Steven Rosen considers vegetarianism in Christianity, Judaism, Islam, Hinduism and Buddhism. The results of his research will come as a surprise to many religious adherents. You'll discover how vegetarianism is an ideal shared by all religions which teach mercy and respect for all creatures.

Diet for Transcendence is the perfect gift for your loved ones or yourself.
Order your copies today!

Available from your local bookseller, or just fill out the order form in back
and fax it, or call us toll free at:
1-888-TORCHLT (867-2458) Fax: (209) 337-2354

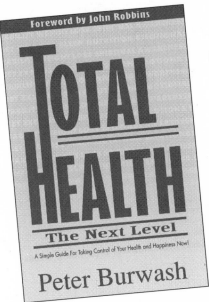

Total Health: The Next Level

A Simple Guide For
Taking Control of Your
Health and Happiness Now!

Exploding the Myths of America's Diet and Exercise Programs

by Peter Burwash
Foreword by John Robbins

$11.95 ISBN #1-887089-10-1
6"x 9", paper 156 pgs.

"Read **Total Health** and heed its wise and compassionate counsel, and you will be well on the way to new levels of aliveness, healing and joy."

John Robbins, Author,
Diet for a New America

Most of us put health and vitality at the top of our goal lists. But we have a hard time achieving it. Despite having so much information at our fingertips and the presence of enormous nutrition, diet and exercise industries enticing us with promises, most of us find remaining committed to a healthy life style a losing battle. Why?

For more than 20 years Peter Burwash has been answering this question and teaching people around the world the simple truths of how to finally reach their goals of health and happiness. He explains with simplicity and compassion how our food and life style choices have a life-changing impact not only on our own future, health and happiness, but that of the entire planet.

Total Health is a wonderful gift for friends, loved ones or yourself.
Order your copies today!

Available from your local bookseller, or just fill out the order form in back
and fax it, or call us toll free at:
1-888-TORCHLT (867-2458) Fax: (209) 337-2354

Book Order Form ────────────

☎ Telephone orders: Call 1-888-TORCHLT (1-888-867-2458).
Have your VISA or MasterCard ready.

✳ FAX orders: 209-337-2354

✉ Postal orders: Torchlight Publishing   PO Box 52
Badger CA 93603-0052 USA

▲ World Wide Web: www.torchlightpub.com

Please send the following: QTY

• **The Vegetarian Revolution**, by Giorgio Cerquetti $14.95 x ___ = $ _____

• **Diet for Transcendence**, by Steven Rosen $11.95 x ___ = $ _____

• **Total Health: The Next Level,** by Peter Burwash $11.95 x ___ = $ _____

                              Sales Tax: (CA residents add 7.75%) . . . .$ _____

                              S/H (see below) . . . .$ _____

TOTAL . . . . $ _____

○ Please send me more information on other books published by Torchlight Publishing.

Company: _____

Name: _____

Address: _____

City:_____ State_____ Zip_____

(I understand that I may return any books for a full refund — for any reason,
no questions asked.)

Payment:

○ Check/money order enclosed   ○ VISA   ○ MasterCard

Card Number: _____

Name on Card: _____ Exp. date_____

Signature: SMYRNA PUBLIC LIBRARY _____

Shipping and handling:

USA : $3.00 for first book and $1.75 for each additional book. Air mail per book (USA only) — $4.00
Canada : $5.00 for first book and $2.50 for each additional book
Foreign countries: $8.00 for first book, $4.00 for each additional book.
Surface shipping may take 3-4 weeks. Foreign orders please allow 6-8 weeks for delivery.